GET A BANGIN' BODY

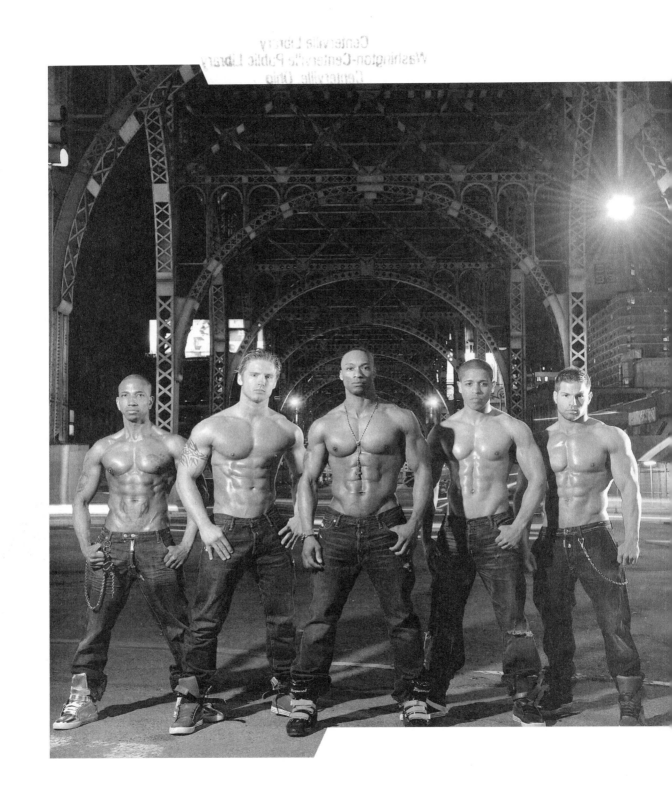

GET A BANGIN' BODY

BODY

THE CITY GYM BOYS'
ULTIMATE BODY WEIGHT WORKOUT
FOR MEN AND WOMEN

CHARLES LaSALLE

WITH PETER RICHMOND

AVERY
A MEMBER OF
PENGUIN GROUP (USA) INC.
NEW YORK

Published by the Penguin Group
Penguin Group (USA) Inc., 375 Hudson Street, New York, New York 10014, USA
Penguin Group (Canada), 90 Eglinton Avenue East, Suite 700, Toronto, Ontario M4P 2Y3, Canada (a division of Pearson Penguin Canada Inc.)
Penguin Books Ltd, 80 Strand, London WC2R 0RL, England
Penguin Ireland, 25 St Stephen's Green, Dublin 2, Ireland (a division of Penguin Books Ltd)
Penguin Group (Australia), 250 Camberwell Road, Camberwell, Victoria 3124, Australia
(a division of Pearson Australia Group Pty Ltd)
Penguin Books India Pvt Ltd, 11 Community Centre, Panchsheel Park, New Delhi–110 017, India
Penguin Group (NZ), 67 Apollo Drive, Rosedale, North Shore 0632, New Zealand (a division of Pearson New Zealand Ltd)
Penguin Books (South Africa) (Pty) Ltd, 24 Sturdee Avenue, Rosebank, Johannesburg 2196, South Africa

Penguin Books Ltd, Registered Offices: 80 Strand, London WC2R 0RL, England

Interior photographs courtesy John Labbe

Most Avery books are available at special quantity discounts for bulk purchase for sales promotions, premiums, fund-raising, and educational needs. Special books or book excerpts also can be created to fit specific needs. For details, write Penguin Group (USA) Inc. Special Markets, 375 Hudson Street, New York, NY 10014.

ISBN 978-1-58333-450-8

Printed in the United States of America
10 9 8 7 6 5 4 3 2 1

Book design by Lovedog Studio

Neither the publisher nor the authors are engaged in rendering professional advice or services to the individual reader. The ideas, procedures, and suggestions contained in this book are not intended as a substitute for consulting with your physician. All matters regarding your health require medical supervision. Neither the authors nor the publisher shall be liable or responsible for any loss or damage allegedly arising from any information or suggestion in this book.

While the authors have made every effort to provide accurate telephone numbers and Internet addresses at the time of publication, neither the publisher nor the authors assume any responsibility for errors, or for changes that occur after publication. Further, the publisher does not have any control over and does not assume any responsibility for author or third-party websites or their content.

ALWAYS LEARNING

PEARSON

"If you want to make any major contribution to society, you have to be at your best, physically and mentally"

CONTENTS

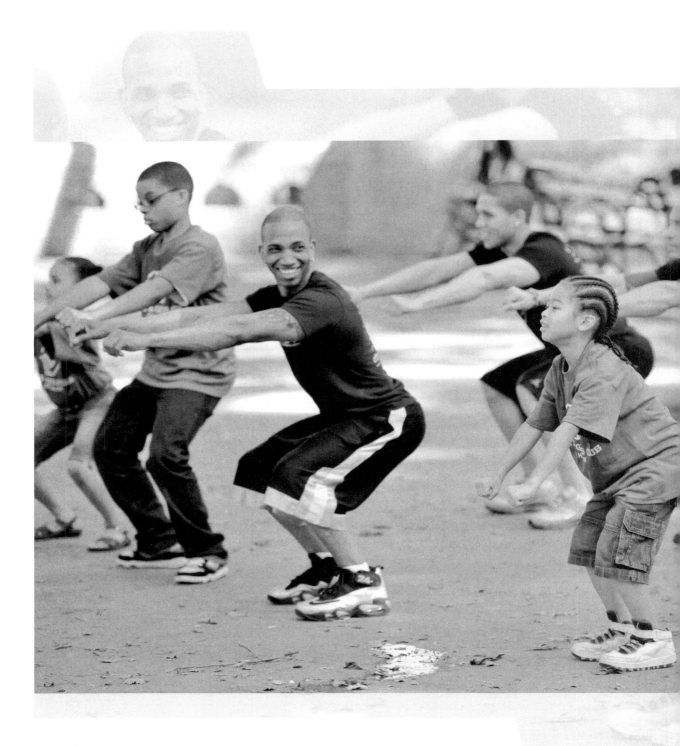

INTRODUCTION

MAYBE I'M STANDING IN THE MIDDLE OF A CIRCLE of kids from the Boys & Girls Club of Harlem, in an open, breezy spot in Jackie Robinson Park, as I do every Friday. It's one of the highlights of my week. The kids really look forward to the workout—especially the overweight ones—because with every hour of jumping jacks, squats and quick feet, they get a little more pride in themselves.

Or maybe Batista and I are in the exercise room at Creative Life-styles, a residential-care facility in the Bronx, where the staff usually directs exercises for the patients. But on this day, we're working with the staff themselves because the executives of this nonprofit want their employees to be fit. After all, it's hard to help others when you're having trouble helping yourself. So we're facing a room full of everyday Americans—Latino, black, white, male, female, young, old—and all with different fitness challenges. We work with them for two hours a week doing lunges, push-ups and jump squats for a few months, and we can see the difference in their bodies and their attitudes.

Or maybe a half dozen of us are in a high school working with Dr. Mehmet Oz's HealthCorps, getting teenagers to realize that obesity isn't nearly as cool as having a six-pack. We might be in the gym or the auditorium or the cafeteria—which is the most fun of all because it's a room where the kids are usually wasting time. But once we start challenging them to follow us and work out, that all changes.

Three different City Gym Boys workouts, and one thing in common: not a single weight or weight machine to be seen anywhere. Every one of these workouts involves nothing but body weight exercises.

Why body weight? Because as you'll see when you read this book, "simple" is our philosophy, whether we're talking about exercise, nutrition or lifestyle. From the time that I founded City Gym Boys fifteen years ago, we have stressed getting back to basics and using the tools that nature has given us to enhance our lives.

That's why we'll never do drugs. That's why, like our hunter-gatherer ancestors of 50,000 years ago, for every calorie we take in, we make sure to work it off. That's called balance—nature's balance. And what could be more natural than using your own body's weight to help you get in shape? What form of resistance could be more in tune with your own body's needs than your own body? It's the perfect counterweight—challenging, and designed just for you.

You wouldn't mind winning a few bodybuilding trophies like us? You want to play professional football? Well, sure—you'll have to hit the weight room. But you wouldn't have picked up this book if you were aiming to be Mr. Olympia.

You picked up this book because you wanted to find a way to get your body in shape and finally realize the potential you've always had.

You picked up this book because you didn't want to resort to a weird diet or a dangerous supplement or a fitness book that required a gym.

You picked up this book because you remembered those school days on the football team or the field hockey team or the basketball team, and the training workouts that were nothing but push-ups and sit-ups and leg lifts—and they worked.

Well, no matter how old you are, who you are, or where you are, body weight exercises are the answer. You can work out any time, any place. Whether in your office, your hotel room, your living room or your backyard, your workout equipment is always with you.

I'm not promising that you'll look exactly like a City Gym Boy after you read this book. That's not the goal. But I can promise that you'll be a better *you*. It's time for you to take control of your body and get the fitness results you've always desired. And notice that I said *your* body—not mine or Markus's or Cisko's or Betty's or Steve's or Klae's. As we start, you don't want to try to accomplish something beyond what you can do; that just sets you up for physical and emotional failure. You're trying to get your best body within your own means. Be true to your own limits. Push them, within your realistic means. That will spell *your* success.

And that's why body weight exercises are perfect for everyone: It's resistance training at its best. Your body has its own natural limits and built-in, achievable goals. Resistance training is, simply, going against gravity. Whether you're using your body as the weight or free weights in a gym, the main benefit of resistance training is muscle building. Now, this isn't quite as obvious as it sounds. Muscle isn't simply something to be used to look good or impress your buddies with your bench presses. Muscle is an integral part of the working system of that body you're about to start working on. Muscle keeps you young. Muscles protect your joints. Mus-

> **"What could be more natural than using your own body's weight to help you get in shape?"**

cle burns more calories. The fatter you are, the slower your body's metabolism. But, the more muscle cells you have, the more fat you're going to burn. Muscle speeds up your metabolism and creates a furnace in your body.

Weight alone isn't the only way to change resistance; you can take your workout to the next level by adjusting the angles in your exercises. Your body needs shock to change, and switching angles of resistance can give you that shock, creating the ripple effect of transforming your body.

"At this point in my life, staying in shape is the only option"

With the simplest strategies, we are going to show you that the key to getting your own bangin' body is as simple as any daily routine in your life—with far more rewarding results. For City Gym Boys, staying fit is all about lifestyle. Once something becomes part of your lifestyle, it's effortless. And once it starts turning your life around, it becomes the focus of your day.

When people see me at festivals, parades or modeling gigs they ask, "How do you do it?" The simple answer is that at this point in my life, staying in shape is the only option. Like eating, hydrating and sleeping, fitness has become a fundamental part of my life.

Body weight workouts have the power to put you in that same place, too, no matter who you are. Maybe you're a housewife with three kids, and after meals, laundry and soccer practice, you can't find the time (or money) to maintain a gym membership. I'll show you how to move the furniture in your living room, throw on some sweats, and get to work—right here, right now.

Maybe you're a college student, stressed out by final exams, trying to keep from reaching for that last sugar doughnut in the box on your desk. You need to clear your mind, but the gym is closed. Well, I'm going to show you what you can do right now in your dorm room to get your blood pumping and your mind working again.

Maybe you're a middle-aged guy, intimidated by the gym and the bangin' bodies all around you (or just your own reflection in the mirrored walls). Fair enough. No one has to see you huff and puff to reach that twentieth push-up when you're doing it in the comfort of your own weight-free bedroom. But huff and puff you should, and huff and puff you will.

Of course, if you can do our body weight workouts anywhere, at any time, that leaves you little room for excuses. But I have a feeling that, by now, you're done with excuses. This time, you're serious about change.

So are we.

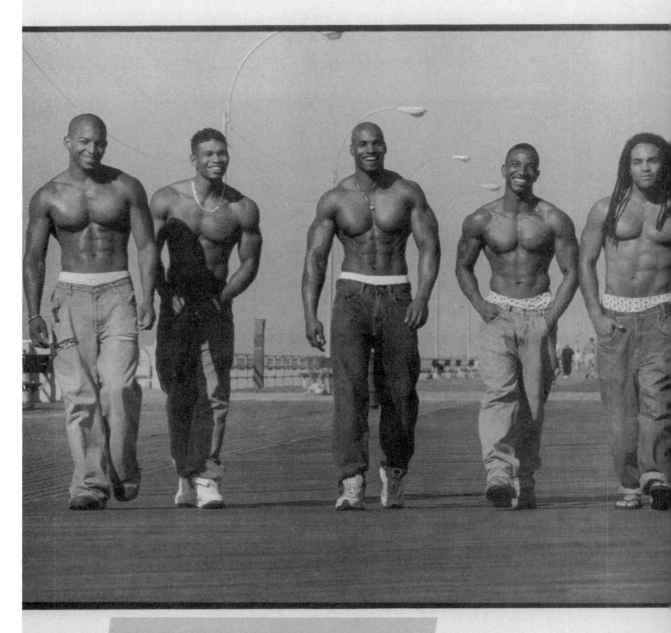

The original City Gym Boys (left to right):
Luis, Flex, Ishmel, Charles and Marshall.
© 1997 Jonathan Atkin

CHAPTER 1

HOW IT ALL BEGAN

THE WEIGHT ROOM AT THE ANCIENT CITY GYM IN lower Manhattan that was called Carmine Recreation Center was cramped and moldy and noisy. It smelled like sweat and old socks. And I loved it.

Carmine Recreation didn't have televisions playing CNN or CNBC or MTV above the treadmills. It didn't serve wheatgrass cocktails at a juice bar. Businessmen didn't store their designer watches in padlocked lockers. Women in leotards didn't watch themselves in mirrors, waiting for their phones to ring.

Carmine Recreation Center was home to regular New Yorkers who couldn't afford fancy gym memberships and who took their workouts seriously. And no one took his workouts as seriously as I did. From my first few days in the gym, sixteen years ago, that century-old brick castle—with its winding, windowless corridors and its tiny running track perched above the noisy, sweaty basketball court—felt like home.

I knew I'd found my place. And I knew I'd found my passion.

I had just started fashion modeling in those days, but that was simply a job for me; it wasn't my purpose. But when I started to work out seriously, I was immediately hooked, because the more I molded my body, the better I started feeling about myself. And while I was changing the way I looked from the outside, I was also changing the inside: A shy kid from Queens who'd been searching for his calling was becoming a man with confidence.

The clang-clank of the weights, and the grunts of the lifters around me became the sound track to my mission. The regulars in the weight room became my supporting cast: "You've got it, little man! Stick with us, little man—we'll show you how. You're a natural!"

And it turned out I was. Before I walked into that city gym, I'd always been active, in fairly good shape. I didn't have a strong physique, because I'd just never trained that hard. I wasn't expected to have a bangin' body, and I never thought I could get one.

But from my very first workout at the city gym, I wasn't cut any slack. "You're going to start training your hardest *right now*," said Luis, a handsome Puerto Rican guy with a model's looks. "No letting up," said Marshall, a light-skinned African-American guy with very long, thick dreads. I had to give them my best. They demanded it.

Now, keep in mind: These guys were hardcore. They didn't pay attention to advertisements in fancy magazines that tried to tell them how to look, what to wear, or what to buy, because they made their own rules. They didn't get brolic (that's New Yorkese for "muscular to the maximum") because it was the macho thing to do. They worked to perfection because it's what made them elite. But unlike

"The more I molded my body, the better I started feeling about myself"

Olympic elite, or NBA elite, their brand of elite is available to anyone who can meet the challenge.

I hadn't been challenging myself. But now, these workouts became a whole lot more interesting. The guys in the city gym showed me what it was like to change my body by challenging myself. Comparing yourself with others is a dead end. But challenging yourself—now, that's the key.

Of course, it was hard to ignore the other challenge: trying to live up to the examples of the guys around me. We were from different backgrounds and cultures, and we had different bodies. But soon we bonded, like a team, and we believed in the same philosophies. We didn't need steroids. We didn't need the status that comes from belonging to the "right" gym (not that we could have afforded it anyway). We knew that there's only one thing you need to get a bangin' body: motivation. The type of motivation that has to come from inside you and you alone.

Having others recognize your work, commitment and sacrifice doesn't hurt, though. A couple of months into my new life, my boys encouraged me to compete in a bodybuilding contest over in the Brownsville neighborhood of Brooklyn—Mike Tyson's old neighborhood.

The gym was dingy. I didn't know how to pose. I didn't know *what* to do. But when I went on stage, I felt . . . good. It felt *right*. And when it was over? First place: Charles LaSalle. I had never won a trophy in my life. It was two feet tall but looked like it was six feet tall to me. I'd never been so proud of myself.

That was a moment—walking home with that trophy—that I'd never had before. I had never had *anything* like that feeling before. The lightbulb had come on: "Bingo. I can change my life." And I have.

If you never get that feeling, you can never truly believe you can lose that weight or gain that muscle. You can't buy that moment. But you can help someone find it. And that's where we come in.

That trophy still stands in my apartment in Washington Heights.

I see it every day. It reminds me of where it all began—and how far I still have to go.

I WAS ON MY WAY. Something had clicked. I began to feed off the *natural* energy of the group. I knew I'd found what I was looking for, and the ego-boost of winning more trophies didn't hurt. But the trophies never meant nearly as much as being part of a brotherhood of guys who knew that exercise is the key to the good life, and that feeling good because you earned it (without crazy scam-artist diets or shortcuts that never work) is as good as life gets.

I'd found a family. I was winning—not just on the stage, but in a whole lot of ways. Now came the question: What to do with my knowledge? How to spread the word to a nation plagued by obesity and diabetes and faddish diets? And then, with a little help from my subconscious, I took the next step.

I'm a huge believer in getting a good night's sleep; it's a big part of any fitness formula. We need as much pure rest as we do pure exercise. When our body is at rest for all the right reasons, our mind follows suit. And on the night of New Year's Eve 1996, I had a dream: I'd put together a group, a fitness group that could reach far and wide. We could train others. And with our distinctive look, we could get some modeling gigs to advance the cause.

We could take our simple message to a culture grown lazy: By changing your body, you're changing your destiny. By shifting the focus from what you eat to what you do, you can turn your life around. And when you turn your own life around, the example leads to exponential change around you. As we travel and teach, the City Gym Boys have seen that firsthand.

All you have to do is want it badly enough. It's that simple.

I hustled to the gym that next day, thinking, "This is it!" But first I had to convince the guys. So I approached Luis. He was immediately all in. "We could make calendars," he said. "We could spread the word by spreading the look." I liked the idea.

But now came the tough part. I wanted to enlist Ishmel: the biggest, strongest guy in the gym. Like Tyson, he had this lisp that somehow made him a little more menacing. When Ishmel wanted to use a weight someone else was using, that guy would give it up without Ishmel's saying a word. He was big, he was brolic and he had a huge, thick neck. But he also had a nice look about him. Ish had a good, steady job, and he'd come into the gym in a suit, take it off and turn into Superman. And you knew he could put a hurting on you if he wanted to.

So, needless to say, I was a little scared. I didn't want him to look down at me and say, "What kind of crazy idea is this?"

We hadn't had a single conversation. I just knew he had a look, and that the group's success would depend on having a variety of different looks. I *did know* that he knew I was legitimate. Everyone in the gym knew that I had won a couple of competitions, so he knew I was on his level.

So I went over, and I dropped my voice, trying to seem cool. "Hey, big man," I said. Inside I'm shaking.

He looks at me: "Whassup?"

"Yo," I said. "I have an idea for a fitness company. A group of us guys get together and we entertain and train people. We'll do calendars and shows. What do you think?"

Ish looked at me for a second, and all I could think was that he was going to say, "Get the hell out of my face!" Instead, he thought for a few seconds, but those seconds stretched into hours before he finally nodded: "Hmm. I'm feeling that. Yes, I'm feeling that." And that was the moment I knew I had the group. If the centerpiece of the gym wanted to be a part of this, it had to be good.

Months later, I got my first personal training job at David Barton Gym, an upscale spot in SoHo—although I still did my workouts at the city gym with my boys. But I started talking to other business people at the SoHo gym and one of my clients, Rich, was a Wall Street kind of guy, so I went to him for business advice. This whole thing was a little out of my league, and I needed some perspective.

> **"All you have to do is want it badly enough"**

> **"We're in it because a beautiful body brings a beautiful mind and spirit"**

I said, "Rich, what do you think of this idea I have: a fitness company with a group of guys who look good, feel good and lead by example. A group that can reach the inner city, where the obesity and diabetes are like a plague."

I thought he'd say, "Do some market research." Instead, he said, "I think you're on to something." Now, Rich is not a guy from the 'hood; he's a middle-aged top executive. So once he gave me the stamp of approval, I said to myself, "This idea is more than a pipe dream: It can be real, and it can be important. We can really do some good. We can really translate our passion into other people. Other people might really want to know how to change their lives . . . and change the world."

That was a sign to me. I realized that our message had the potential to reach a culture that desperately needed to hear it and persuade people to get off the couch and *move.*

WHEN I MEET PEOPLE I want to introduce fitness to—personal training clients, potential City Gym Boys, friends who reach out to me for help and advice—it's always kind of like a first date. You have to find a way to reach them. All these doubts and fears and insecurities come in: "Well, I don't really like working out. I don't like the gym scene. Is my body going to change?"

But then, if they follow my advice, sooner or later they're waking up in the morning and texting me saying, "When can we train again? How soon?" Then I meet them at the gym, and I see it in their face: They've got the bug. They're hooked! And from that moment on, my job is done. They're a new person. And those are always the most satisfying moments in my life.

So now I had the group. I had a way to make a difference. I was a little nervous at the beginning, but as soon as the group started to come together, I knew I'd be good at leading. I'd never been a leader before, because I'd never been confident that I was the master of anything. Now, I knew I was qualified to be in command.

Maybe this is the way that all good coaches and leaders feel: ready to lead a group toward a better place. All I know is that it now feels natural.

AND WHAT WOULD WE be called? That was easy. We moved up to Twenty-third Street, to the Asser Levy Recreation Center. Asser Levy was a big step up, an ornate old bathhouse with plenty of space in the weight room—and that same comforting, funky old smell. It was classier, but it was still a city gym.

And one day this particular girl had taken a liking to us, as the girls tend to do. She saw us working out as always, and she laughed and said, "You and your boys are the City Gym Boys. Because you're always in the damned gym!"

The City Gym Boys: That said it all. And that's how it started.

Before long, we had our first calendar and modeling gig. Today we're two dozen strong: a group of natural bodybuilders from every walk of life. I look at us like a professional sports team with an active roster each season of twenty to twenty-four. For some events, I have my top five; for the calendar, I choose the top fourteen. I'm something like a player and a coach.

Do we have competitions within the group? Yes. Do some of the guys work harder to get to the top level of the group? Yes. (And yes, I'm in charge. It's my way or the highway when it comes to the rules of being a City Gym Boy.)

The bottom line is that our message is obviously reaching people who want to hear our ideas. We've worked with Dr. Mehmet Oz's HealthCorps, the American Diabetes Association, and even McDonald's. We've worked with First Lady Michelle Obama's Let's Move! initiative. Our events have drawn the likes of Lil' Kim, Usher and Jennifer Hudson.

But we're not in it for the collective ego; we're in it because the higher our profile, the more good we can do. That's the honest truth. You'll see: When you get your own bangin' body, sure, you're going to want to show it off. But you're also going to want to spread the word of your fitness journey.

We're in it because a beautiful body brings a beautiful mind and spirit. And if you're looking for that combination, we're all united in the belief that movement and motion are they keys to getting us there. So you'll find us in inner-city high schools and in rural elementary schools. You'll find us at ethnic festivals all over NYC, walking the walk and preaching our motto: It's not what you eat, it's what you do.

That's our mantra, and that's how this book is going to change your life.

" Effort is everything "

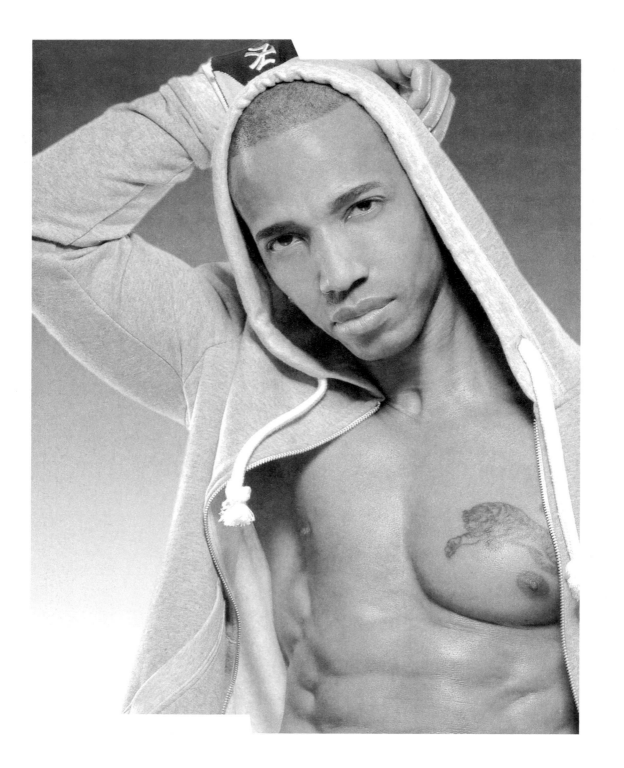

MY WAKE-UP CALL

DEEP DOWN, I ALWAYS WANTED TO BE IN SHOW BUSIness—probably a way for a shy kid to express himself. As one of many siblings, I always kind of felt like I didn't have anything to say when everyone else was talking a lot. So I just sort of watched the world around me, waiting for my calling. Waiting for something to reach out and grab me.

In high school I was a quiet, slightly nerdy, honors student, and the only thing that kind of made me hip was how stylishly I dressed. So one day, some of the girls in my school said, "Charles, you dress so nice. You have to be in this year's annual school fashion show."

"I'm not a model," I said.

MY **WAKE-UP** CALL　17

"But it's a chance to show off your clothes," they replied. "It'll be fun."

So I figured, "Why not?" and agreed to participate in the fashion show about three weeks later.

The night of the show was upon me and I was excited, anxious and nervous. Before that night, I always thought it would be scary to be on stage in the spotlight, but when it was my turn to walk down the runway my fears vanished. I looked out at that crowd, let the applause wash over me and thought, maybe for the first time in my life, "I'm in control. I'm the *man!*" Suddenly, I knew I could do this.

Of course, then I wanted to be in other fashion shows: church, neighborhood, anywhere. At the other shows I met people who had the same interests as I did, and they led me to shows in Manhattan. Once I was in Manhattan, my ambitions grew to encompass the whole showbiz world. I began to think I could really be a model or a dancer or an actor. I'd found my people. I'd found my place.

It's not that I wasn't close with my family. But my brothers and sisters didn't take show business seriously. This was a large blue-collar family, with blue-collar values. My dad's Cuban, my mom's Jamaican, and as with many emigrant parents, their main goal for their children was for them to get an education. Anything else was a distraction. There was no room for a career in entertainment in my parent's idea of the American Dream—but there was in mine.

But the biggest challenge that I faced in realizing my dream of being a successful model was my height. At five feet, nine inches, I was lost in the shadow of the other models. In the modeling business, you can't get much serious work unless you're six feet, minimum. So I started to concentrate on acting classes. But I was attending college full-time, too. I had to take night classes and juggle the two lives. I wanted to break into the business, to find a way to recapture that feeling I'd had when I took the stage back in high school. I had some gigs, but it was mostly minor modeling, and I had to sneak it in on weekends, when I wasn't taking classes.

I was no supermodel. I didn't know if I was really an actor, either; I wasn't feeling the passion. I had the feeling that somewhere along the line, maybe this wasn't my true calling. That's when life-changing moment No. 2 occurred, when my sheltered life changed, and my eyes were opened wide: in, of all places, Cape Town.

When I look back, it's sort of funny that things started to turn around for me not in some famous modeling capital like Paris or London but in a city way off the fashion map. It seems fitting that my trip to a country that had just officially stopped discriminating against blacks would lead to my forming a group that's trying to empower people of color, and do what it can to raise the health consciousness and inner confidence of people in the inner cities.

IN THE LATE NINETIES, South Africa was the hottest fashion market for new models. White female models could work everywhere, but black male models couldn't. Apartheid had been lifted, so South Africa was finally opened up to the world politically and artistically. Now, I'll admit: I wasn't very socially conscious.

Running around the streets of New York, you'd hear models say, "I'm going to Paris, Milan, London." But all of a sudden you started hearing a lot of black guys saying, "South Africa. They're hiring!" Even if we were not politically conscious, we got pulled in.

I've always loved traveling, so I jumped at the opportunity to do so. I did a little research and found an agency in Cape Town. I faked my height. I was able to get a few advance bookings, which is always an advantage, so I'd have a little money to live on.

I got a three-month visa, and there I was, in the new modeling frontier for black models. I got a room in a house that rented to models. There were eight to ten models coming and going every week, and it was totally hectic. It was sort of like MTV's *Real World*, except it didn't feel real at all. There was a dreamy aspect of it all because it was so foreign—and so beautiful. It was like living in a little paradise.

My roommate and I decided to escape the house and get our own place—a small house with a view of beautiful Table Mountain. And I got some work. I put lifts in my shoes for a shoot for a high-fashion magazine, but I was still a few inches shorter than the other model. The photographer managed to pose us in such a way that we looked like we were the same height, and the spread turned out great.

I even landed a coveted *cover* of a magazine. Not a black magazine, either—a national magazine. For a black guy to make the cover of a South African general-interest magazine back then was a big deal. My friends were surprised and excited for me: This guy from New York City—who wasn't even six feet tall—was going to get a cover that would be in the supermarkets.

I guess I had a pretty good look. But as the days went on in this enchanted land, I cared less about the modeling and more about the culture and the experience. Soon, I didn't care about the modeling at all. I fell in love with the people. I saw poverty, and I saw homeless kids. I saw the street kids. And the most amazing thing of all was that these people, who had nothing, were so happy. They considered every day a gift. They didn't expect favors or luxury or material pleasures.

Every day when I woke, I didn't want to go to photo shoots or hustle up work; I just wanted to go walk on the streets with these people. I began to start feeling that everything I'd been looking for—money, fame, modeling, acting—just wasn't enough. Suddenly, none of those things seemed important.

The modeling, the lifts in my shoes and the trick photography—that was all illusion. The South African street kids, smiling and dancing and holding hands even though they had no money—that was real.

I was supposed to go home after three months, but I managed to get my visa extended another three months. I didn't want to leave. I could feel it—a spiritual change was happening. For the first time, I was away from all the old influences, all the old advice, all the old pressures and uncertainties. I came to realize that I never had a true passion for the modeling and the acting. The head shots, auditions and rejections just weren't for me.

Even landing gigs wasn't all that meaningful anymore. It helped boost my ego, and occasionally my bank account, but it wasn't as if I loved it. I loved the idea of what all of it might get me, but I didn't love the process.

I *so* wanted to do something I loved to do, but by now I had no idea what that would be. I did know this: I'd never been happier than when I was on the streets with the street kids of South Africa. I'd see them all over the city, mainly during the daytime. You would not see them sleeping on the streets. And I always wondered where they'd go at night. Their spirit was so amazing. I'd wonder, *What are they celebrating?* Their smiles lit up my day. They had no real place to go, but their family was the people on the streets.

And they made me start to realize that trying to be a star was a useless road to travel. Materialistically, these people had nothing compared with what I had back in the States, but here they were— making me happy! They were laughing, they were dancing, and their message was clear: Enjoy life and live it to the fullest. I knew that when I came back home, I would really start doing what was giving me pleasure. I knew I had to start over, get back to basics.

Something else struck me about the Cape Town city kids: They were all in excellent shape from their moving and dancing, running and singing. Not one of them was overweight. When I returned home to the States, I was a different man.

> "*I could feel it—a spiritual change was happening*"

IF WE'RE LUCKY, we all reach a point in our lives when we realize that success doesn't equal money or ego gratification. We reach a turning point; and after spending time in South Africa, I had reached mine. Betty Peralta reached hers on the day she realized that even though she was fit enough to make anyone envious, she wasn't being everything she could be. She had to raise the bar. She had to find a trainer who would make her challenge herself to reach her utmost capabilities. She wanted to take her body to the next level.

Betty had attended a few abs-workout classes I led, and the intensity of the workouts had pulled her in. Betty loves to be challenged in her workouts, and it just so happened that her then boyfriend (now her husband) was one of my old friends from the neighborhood.

"I want him to train me," she told my friend. So he asked me if I would, and I happily obliged. I remembered her from my class as a hard, devoted worker (and the obvious: as very pretty). He wanted her to be pushed as much as she wanted to be pushed.

Betty is a beautiful, feminine woman. She's a mother of two young children, she's an elementary school teacher, and she trains just like one of the guys. She does squats. She does resistance training. She does cardio. Like any woman, Betty has the constant challenge to burn body fat—those are the genetics that she and every woman deal with.

And every day, between her job and her family, she rises to the challenge. She's as amazing a role model as you're ever going to find.

BETTY PERALTA

I teach children with special needs at the Amistad Dual Language School in northern Manhattan, a highly regarded institution with a reputation for excellence. I make a living by working with students with very different conditions and needs. I am also a wife and a mother of two very active boys—a one-year-old and a three-year-old—and I'm always aware that they each have different ways of learning and growing.

So while the City Gym Boys can give you guidance about fitness and offer a body weight regimen that caters to your general level of fitness and experience, you have to find your own level, your own realistic goals and your own way of meeting them.

If you're going to take the next step, the way I did, workouts have to be a part of the day you really look forward to. So you have to find a way of taking the City Gym Boys' message and making it work for you. Everyone's fitness goals are different: Some of us want perfect legs or a six-pack, while some of us just want to get rid of fat. But the way I see it, we all share one goal: getting to the place where we feel good about ourselves. And Charles teaches—and lives by the idea—that the way to feel good about yourself is to be as healthy as you can be.

WITH CHARLES, I knew I'd found the right trainer. He's a very positive person, and he made it easy for me to work even harder than I already was. Then, in a way, I'd been heading for this kind of fitness routine for a long time. I was a tomboy as a child. So, I have always been a very physically active person. In later years, my husband, Joel, then my best friend, introduced me to a book he was reading. And when I picked up Bill Phillips's *Body for Life* and read it cover to cover, it changed my life. The book talked about "gym rats," and I recognized myself. I was eighteen, and I was going to the gym three, four times a week. Same routines. Same weights. But my body had hit a plateau.

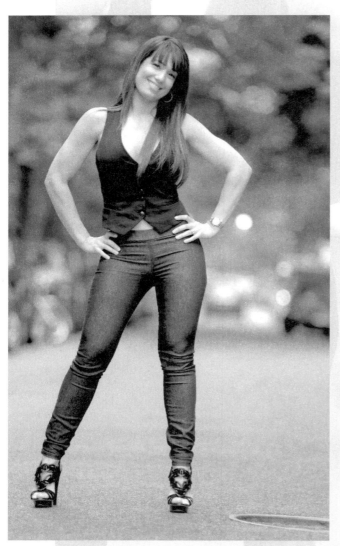

I wanted to take it higher. It's all really just about wanting it, and when you want the things that you really need—like health, fitness and self-esteem—the road is never going to be easy. You have to be into it. You have to have the discipline to say, "I have to go work out" on a consistent basis. Making a commitment to making yourself better is not a part-time thing.

For instance, maybe after a winter of working out, you say, "I'm done now. I look good. I can support this body for the rest of the summer." For many people, the summer is the time when it's hard to say no to how much you want to eat, and it's even harder to do the work your body knows it needs to burn off those additional calories.

So maybe you say, "Now I can have fun, and I'll get back to my workouts in the fall." No! We're talking about a lifestyle change. If you're ready to make a full-time commitment to changing your body you have to make a full-time commitment to changing your lifestyle.

But change is not a cookie cutter thing. Everyone's starting point is different, so evaluate yourself. If you hate being confined to the gym, take your workout outdoors. No matter where you prefer to move your body, just make sure to give it your best shot every time.

But if you're a woman, don't stay away from resistance training. Some women are so scared to use weights: "I'll look like a man!" But they wouldn't think that way if they were educated about achieving and maintaining fitness. Resistance training, whether with body weight or gym weights, builds muscle, which allows you to burn fat. For women to get a toned body, resistance training, combined with a good cardio regimen is the way to go. You'll be fit, you'll look good and you'll feel so much better.

You will also sleep better and have more energy, and you won't focus on food as much. When you're exercising and feeling good about yourself, food becomes less important to you.

And when you do eat what you want to eat, have the discipline not to eat too much and to burn it off afterward. It's fine to have the fried dough and the ice cream once in a while, but moderation is the key. The unfortunate truth is that there are people who simply can't afford to buy "healthy foods" even if they wanted to. We all know that. As a mother, I can tell you from firsthand experience: So-called healthy foods are expensive! Every time you want to shop for the organic stuff, it's a pretty penny.

But that doesn't mean you should just shrug your shoulders and say, "I can't afford to be healthy and look good." It's not so much about what you eat; it's about what you do to burn it off. I know it's tempting to think, "Who has the time to exercise or take it to the next workout level, as you did? I have so much more to get done in my day-to-day life."

True, life throws you curveballs, and sometimes things get in the way of the goals we set for ourselves. But don't give up when things don't happen as you plan—just do the best you can.

In the same way, if you set realistic fitness goals and then do everything that you can to achieve them—give it your absolute best, and let nothing get in the way—then those other life goals are going to be easier to achieve as well.

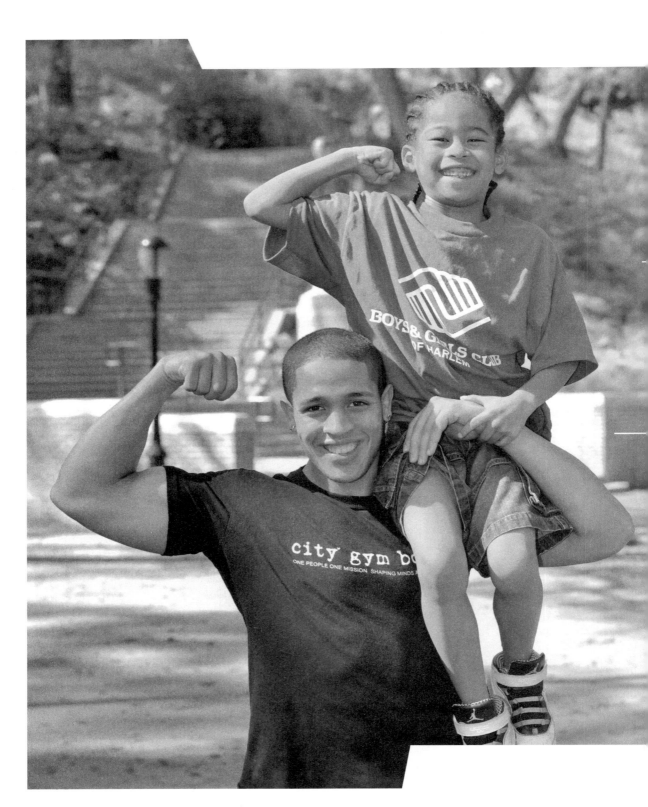

CHAPTER 3

THE BIG ISSUE AT HAND

LET'S DEAL WITH THE REAL ISSUE, THE QUESTION that lies behind the reason we wrote this book: Why are we getting fatter and fatter as a nation? How did we get to a point where more than 60 percent of the nation is overweight? Where the average woman weighs 164 pounds? Where, among children born after 2000, one in three will develop type 2 adult-onset diabetes?

The numbers are scary enough, but you don't need statistics to see the plague. All you have to do is look at the person straining to fit into the seat next to you on the airplane or standing in front of you in the grocery store to know that even as the nation pretends to be growing more health-conscious by going green and organic, something has gone terribly wrong. And it's this: We are obsessed with the idea that food determines our weight. And until we identify the real problem, we're never going to be healthy. As long as we continue to believe that food is going to determine our destiny, we'll be stuck in this rut.

The single greatest contributor to America's sorest shame is that we're a nation that no longer moves. Our children are attached to their video screens. We take the escalator instead of climbing the stairs. We take the crosstown bus instead of walking through the park. We drive a half mile to the drugstore.

We don't leave the house to visit our friends in person; we text them. We don't even go to the office; we can work at home. And when we do go into the office, we're growing even fatter. The workplace is a contributor to obesity. Fifty years ago, half of us worked at jobs that required physical activity. Then manufacturing and farming began to die off. Today, just *one-fifth* of us work at jobs that require physical activity. That indolence is costing the average American 140 calories a day.

Obesity is defined as being more than thirty pounds above a healthy weight, and it's estimated that one in three Americans is obese. That weight is loading down a lot more than just the men, women, boys and girls who are afflicted. It's bringing down an entire nation—economically and emotionally.

> **"The rest of the world is laughing at us for being obese"**

BUT THE GOOD NEWS is that if you enhance your self-esteem by getting into shape, you'll have less stress on a daily basis, and you'll be a whole lot more productive. Now think of the overall effect—on the economy, the community and the nation—if all of us took our lives into our own hands. The rest of the world is laughing at us for being obese, and that's bad enough. Moreover, obesity prevents us from performing at maximum capacity, and that brings us down, too.

Economically, obesity is costing the taxpayer $150 billion a year in medical costs, and another $80 billion in lost productivity. At the rate we're growing, though, that number will be $350 billion in six years—it will account for more than one-fifth of all health-care costs. The state-by-state breakdown of obesity rates, not surprisingly, shows that the poorest states in the country are the fattest. And since the obese are likelier to suffer in the job market, the prospects of those poor states are worsening. It's been documented that overweight people are viewed as less capable by prospective employers. And according to an exhaustive survey of 10,000 people by three sociologists from Utah State and Arizona State University, an overweight woman is at a distinct disadvantage when it comes to education and job prospects.

Do you want to know the most depressing statistic of all? Despite the fact that two out of three Americans are overweight, nine out of ten of us say we have a healthy diet.

We're not fooling anyone but ourselves.

Statistics about how many of us think we're working out enough? Those aren't available. Like so many of the country, academics still think that the problem is caused by our eating habits. Even the academics who study obesity are missing the point.

HOW DID WE GET HERE?

How did it happen? That's an easy, quick history lesson. Sixty years ago, the average American weighed twenty pounds less than he or she does now. And then, what happened sixty years ago? Television established its footing.

For the previous thirty years, radio had captured our imagination, but it had never taken us out of the fields and yards; its comedies and dramas were a reward for a day's hard work. When television began to give us pictures along with words and songs, we gave in: It was so much easier to sit back and let interesting things come to you than go out and find them, especially while enjoying TV dinners.

No, watching a baseball game wasn't quite as much fun as playing in a league with your buddies, but the advantage of watching one was that you could drink a beer and cheer without paying for a ticket. No, watching a funny TV show wasn't as entertaining as a night on the town, but it took less effort.

But even then, we still had a shot at being a responsibly fit culture—until cable came in, and we turned the corner. We outsmarted ourselves. We invented a technology that allowed television to go from five channels to fifty to five hundred.

The next thing we knew, little kids weren't spending summer nights playing stickball on St. Nicholas Avenue or kicking the soccer ball at the school field in the suburbs. They were watching television. By the time the video games showed up, they were already hooked by the hypnotic screen.

And when the Internet took over, well, the idea of any generation finding its joy in life by being active was so alien that the only activity that could get the average kid out of his bedroom was to bike to his best friend's house—to play the next hot video game.

The other day, I saw a couple of kids throwing a football on a street, and I was surprised. That used to happen every day back in my neighborhood. How disappointing is it that seeing kids outside doing some sort of physical activity strikes you as strange? How far out of whack have we become when so many of our *kids* are obese? Childhood is supposed to be the time of unrestrained running, skating, climbing and playing. Today, in my city, the jungle gyms and slides are disappearing from the playgrounds, victims of overconcerned parents.

Obesity is also occurring at a disproportionately high rate in minority communities, especially among Hispanics and African-Americans, which basically dooms our inner-city kids from the start. If a parent is obese, there's a 50 percent chance their child will be, too. Right now, one in five kids is obese—and it's getting worse.

Sadly, the higher the number of fat children grows, the less incentive they have to get rid of the pounds. They may feel bad about themselves, but at least they feel bad together. They reinforce one another, hoping that their collective suffering will make them feel okay about being fat.

And by the way: Being politically correct about this is a disservice to a lot of people. You hear it all the time: "I look good at this weight." Or, "It's okay for somebody to be kind of overweight. She looks good at that size. Not everybody's born to be slim." Or, "I love being fat . . . I love my size . . . Accept me . . . I've always been this way . . . I have big bones in my family." Whatever.

We're humans. We need social approval, and that's a reality. People say it doesn't matter that they're fifty pounds overweight? It's a lie. We *all* want to matter to society, to count. But when you're obese, you don't matter; you don't count. (Or, at least, that's how society makes it seem.)

I see it all the time. There's that nameless overweight girl on the subway who can hardly fit in the seat. Her embarrassment and low self-esteem are evident in her body language. She has a beautiful face, but she doesn't *feel* beautiful, and it's eating her up inside.

But these feelings of "I'm not good enough" are not reserved only for everyday people. Even celebrities can struggle with their self-image because of being overweight. For example, a few years back I was at an event and had the pleasure of meeting a well-known Oscar- and Grammy-winning singer and actress. At the time, she was overweight and, despite being such an incredible talent and having just starred in one of the biggest movies of the year, she still seemed so insecure. She took photos with the guys and me, and her spirit felt so low. It was almost as if she was thinking, "Yeah, I'm the fat girl." I couldn't believe it! I thought to myself, "You have one of the most amazing voices in the world. You should be more confident!"

But over the past year she's lost a lot of weight, and I can see the difference in her self-esteem. She's slimmer, smiling and visibly

"**What happened sixty years ago? Television established its footing**"

more confident. It's as if her spirit has finally come out. And that's what being fit does.

ON ANOTHER LEVEL, obesity has serious societal and cultural implications. What we're talking about here, and what we're trying to do, is so much bigger than people seem to realize. When a society takes its future into its own hands, change becomes more than possible: It becomes attainable, and then it becomes an actual goal.

Right now, we as a society are wallowing in failure as our next generations grow unhealthier and become victims to a disease that used to be nothing but a geriatric ailment: diabetes mellitus. Diabetes is a disease caused by the body's inability to produce sufficient insulin needed in order to regulate blood sugar.

Diabetes has become so ubiquitous that the supermarket magazine racks now feature *Diabetic Living* and *Diabetic Cooking*! The disease is suffered by 21 million Americans, but that number doesn't begin to suggest the really scary part: The number of Americans living with diabetes has almost doubled in the last decade. More than 80 percent of that increase is in type 2 adult-onset diabetes, and 80 percent of type 2 diabetics are obese or overweight.

Fifteen years ago type 2 diabetes was an adult disease. Now, tens of thousands of kids have it—and far more are at risk. The risk is greatest in African-Americans and Hispanics, and the link between obesity and type 2 diabetes is now indisputable.

The cost? A diabetic's annual health-care costs average $13,243—*five times* that of an individual without the disease. Diabetes ranks as the third-highest risk for employers behind heart disease and hypertension (which accounts for the growing number of diabetics who are being fired from their jobs for their condition). The problem is so widespread that a whole new branch of discrimination law has blossomed to defend sufferers of diabetes.

SCHOOL DAZE

It's no surprise that the path to obesity starts early, in elementary and high school, where fat girls are more stigmatized than fat boys, leading to a depressing statistic: Overweight women are less likely to earn college degrees. They also have fewer friends, fewer jobs and lower self-esteem.

While the glass ceiling is being shattered for the healthy population of women, the barriers remain for the obese. The psychological damage from childhood and adolescent obesity can be as damaging as the physical toll that it takes.

But the cost of obesity in high school goes way beyond just the physical and psychological damage. Today, 40 percent of high school students are overweight or obese, which means that two in every five kids aren't at their optimum learning level. But at a time when the United States has fallen dangerously behind the rest of the world in education, we can hardly afford to have kids falling further behind because of something we can fix.

But it's not going to be easy, as I and the rest of the City Gym Boys know well. And when we visit high schools, it's not the girls who are the problem—it's the guys. The girls are instantly drawn to us. As soon as we hit the stage, the girls flock right up there to see what we're all about, to hear our message. The girls don't have the social stigma about working out. It's not unfeminine to look good.

The boys are a much tougher nut to crack. I'll have to pull them over and confront them: "Hey, do you know how to do a push-up?" Some do, but some don't. It takes a little convincing. "Hey," I'll say to the boys, "we're having a competition here. Get your boys over here and see who can do the most push-ups." Once you make them see it as a competition, convincing them that wanting to look fit isn't nerdy or geeky (especially when so many of their entertainment role models are so large) gets a little easier.

"It's not cool to be out of shape," I'll tell them. "You're in high school, and you're telling me you can't do ten push-ups? You're going to be more active, starting right now."

One day working with Dr. Oz's HealthCorps at a high school in the Bronx, one kid watched us do our routine up on stage: getting kids to do push-ups, working out ourselves, putting on a show so that we can teach by example. After all, our best advertisement is our bodies. One six-pack can speak a thousand words.

I could tell from the look in his eye that he thought what we were doing was interesting. So I said, "You want to come over and compete with your classmates in the push-ups contest?"

He said, "I just worked out, so I'm kind of sore." But he kept watching. I knew he wanted to be part of it, because he was watching the way the girls were reacting. I eventually talked him into competing and he went against one of his classmates and won. As a prize, I gave him a City Gym Boys T-shirt.

"Who are you guys?" he said. I handed him my business card.

"Take it home," I said. "Show it to your parents. If they think it's cool for you, give me a call."

That night he called. "My mom says it's cool," he said. "How can I get to be part of it?"

I told him, "I'm going to show you the world of fitness, but this is the deal: You have to go to college. He wanted to get a full-time job after high school, so he could help his family out financially. I told him, "You go to college, I'll help you get part-time work on the side as a personal trainer, and in the end, you'll do a whole lot more for your family than you would if you do not get a college education."

Today, Felix is a proud member of City Gym Boys and is in his first year in college.

WHY DO WE SPEND so much time in the schools? Because adolescence is tough. High school is rough. Thirteen to seventeen is a very trying period: the years when we try to find ourselves and try desperately to fit in. This makes it all the more important for teenagers to feel good about themselves. Working with the high school kids is the most amazing feeling, because once they get their first taste of fitness, you really see a change in their mind-set. The world is no longer an intimidating place: It's a stage to strut with pride.

Here's the goal: to get to the point where working out is cool. And to get there, we have to move beyond the old way of thinking of exercising as a chore. It has to become a fun part of the day.

And with every newly fit adult around them, kids are given another health role model. One of the most satisfying things we've done in the last few years has been working with the mothers of students at George Washington High School in the Washington Heights neighborhood of Manhattan. To reach the students, we've worked with their parents in a ten-week program organized by Dr. Oz's HealthCorps.

It's important for parents to lead by example, but it's hard for a parent to teach the value of fitness and exercise to their children when they are overweight themselves. *Do as I say, not as I do*, doesn't work when it comes to fitness and exercise.

At the G. W. High boot camp, we worked with mothers who hadn't done any exercise in years and who committed to this program because they realized that there was a communication problem. Their kid thinks, "You're fat, you're lazy, so it must be okay for me to be overweight, too." No parent wants his or her child to be a smoker or a drinker or a drug user, but how are you going to get him to a gym when he's never seen you do as much as a sit-up?

"But I don't have the time," the parents will say.

"Yes, you do," we tell them. "While the food is cooking, you do the exercises. While the laundry is drying, you do the exercises. While you're watching TV, you *do the exercises*."

And the results? Soon, their stomachs were sore, and they could feel their butt muscles, and you could see the lightbulbs turning on. And you can bet that their own commitment influenced their kids' commitment.

"You're in high school, and you're telling me you can't do ten push-ups?"

But it's not easy. In his or her own mind, the tenth grader is immortal. But try putting it in perspective for your child. Ask them, "Do you want to be in high school and have to get insulin? Do you want to be bothered with checking your blood sugar every day? Is it cool to have to carry an insulin pump?" If we don't deal with exercise and physical activity in every household and every school from the ground up, weight-related health problems will continue to plague us.

WE WORK IN COLLEGES, too, for a very specific reason: Today's college student experiences a whole new set of anxieties upon entering the world of academia. With the threat of college loan debt coupled with dismal postgraduation job prospects, college students have never been more underprepared to handle the upcoming stresses of university life.

On a tour of five historically black colleges where the City Gym Boys had been enlisted to teach a little fitness to the next generation, I saw it myself: kids who have overcome all the anxieties of adolescence only to panic at the demands of higher education.

But don't take my word for it. For the last quarter of a century, UCLA's Higher Education Research Institute has conducted a comprehensive poll of incoming college freshmen to find out what that next generation is thinking and feeling. It's considered the gold standard of information about this generation's mind-set.

And what did their survey of the 200,000 members of the incoming freshman class of 2010 reveal? That the emotional health of incoming freshmen in America has never been lower. That half of the kids going into college considered themselves "below average" in mental health.

WHEN I WAS IN COLLEGE studying for a test, I'd always get to the point where I couldn't take in any more information. Nothing else was going to go in. My brain would shut down, fried like an overloaded computer.

The solution was easy: Drop the book, go to the gym, and work out—a good, thorough workout where I'd physically break my body down. Then, when I got back to my room, it was as if I'd shut down my brain, rebooted it, and got it firing back up again on all cylinders.

The same can work for you. If you find yourself up at 3:00 a.m. studying for an exam, Shakespeare doesn't make sense anymore and the gym is closed, I suggest you close the book, push back the couch and do your body weight exercise of choice. It'll work wonders for your mind and body.

FOOD SHOULDN'T BE THE FOCUS

How is it that a nation obsessed with diet and nutrition is the fattest nation in the world? We must be doing something very wrong. And we are. As I'm reminded every day, we're focusing on the wrong thing: what we eat.

In New York City, Mount Sinai is one of our best hospitals. As I write this, the hospital has just posted a series of banners outside its main building, which are visible as commuter trains in the city race into the tunnel on their way to Grand Central: "Eat colorful veggies," says one. "Eat fewer sugary snacks," says another. Not a single one says, "Be more active."

It's time to get moving. Literally.

THERE ARE DOZENS of fitness and nutrition books out there; why should the City Gym Boys guide your journey? Why should my guys be the team that sets an example for you? Because this is a very special group of men. We were drawn together by our mutual determination to change our own lives, and now we do whatever we can to change the lives of others. That's powerful stuff. That's a bond that cannot be broken. And hopefully, we'll draw you in to that bond also, because there's strength in numbers. A group is always stronger than the sum of its parts, and when you've made the decision to change your body, support is a good thing to have.

From here on out, you're part of a pretty strong support group: a group that's together because we *want* to be together. We're at the gym at any hour of the day or night because we *want* to be there. We could spend our late nights at a nightclub or a bar. But instead, you'll find us working out in the gym at one o'clock in the morning. (We all have a special fondness for the late-night workout; it's *me* time. It's a great way to end the day, it leads to real sleep, and it gives the next day a great place to start.)

Of course, that's not the kind of training we're recommending to you in these pages. True, by the time you finish this book, some of you may be so hooked that you'll be joining us in the wee hours. But for beginner and intermediate level readers, our goal is simple: We're here to help you turn your life around.

> **"We're focusing on the wrong thing: what we eat"**

IT'S THE OLD-FASHIONED WAY, and it works. Move your body. Do the push-ups while you're waiting for the dinner to cook. Jog to the store. This type of commitment works, and it works for everyone. And let's be clear on one thing from the start: This book is for everyone. And I mean *everyone*. Everyone can create his or her own bangin' body. Everyone has the potential.

Of course, my body is going to look a little different than yours, so don't look at me and shrug your shoulders and say, "I could never look like that." Well, of course not. We're all different. We all have different genetics and different lifestyles.

But "bangin' body" is a relative term. What if you weigh two hundred pounds, you adopt our body weight workout plan, you lose five pounds, and they stay off? You're bangin'.

What if your husband notices that you're looking a little better? You're bangin'.

What if you still have no trace of a six-pack, but that extra layer of fat is shrinking and your love handles are disappearing? You'll begin to see yourself in a new way and, you guessed it—you'll be bangin'.

IF YOU'RE HERE BECAUSE you want to get a better body, and reap all the emotional and mental rewards that come with it, you've come to the right place. In my eyes, nothing else about you matters. *Nothing*. Size, weight, age, sex—it makes no difference to me. Just do the exercises, believe in the City Gym Boys message, and we'll get you where you want to go.

All I need to know about you is that your doctor says you can do the workout. That you're willing. And that you're ready.

Let's be clear: Working out has nothing to do with age, sex, sexuality, ethnicity or culture. Either you want to get a bangin' body, and you want it now, or you don't. Period. End of discussion.

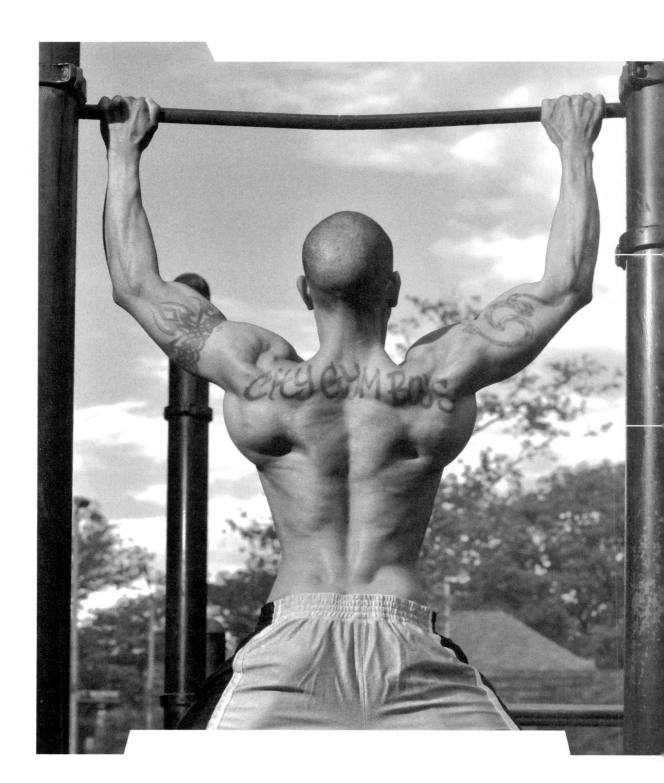

IT'S NOT WHAT YOU EAT, IT'S WHAT YOU DO

CHAPTER 4

I'LL NEVER FORGET A SCENE IN THE ATLANTA AIR-
port a few years ago. The City Gym Boys were on our way
to the *Essence* Music Festival in New Orleans, and we were
walking around the terminal, trying to find a place to eat. Everyone
was looking great and, as usual, people were stopping and looking at
us—who *are* those guys?

So we go into McDonald's, get in line and now people are looking at us in a different way: You guys actually *eat* this stuff?

Well, of course we eat this stuff. I *love* my McDonald's french fries.

The people that we encountered were like just about every other misinformed American out there. They're thinking, "Those guys look amazing. They can't possibly eat fast food. They probably can't eat anything! Wow, what a sacrifice to have to live on broccoli, sprouts, and skinless chicken."

Wow, what a misconception. Sure, food is a factor in the way your body looks and feels. Is it a big factor? No. Does the constant, overwhelming, obsessed media blitz about diets and calories have a place in a society trying to shed its fat? No.

Can you really eat what you want and still have the six-pack? Of course. The fact is, most of the City Gym Boys are young, and many are from the inner city, so the chains have been part of their lives. It would be hypocritical to say, "We don't eat fast food!" when most of the guys do.

Face it: Despite our trend toward locally sourced, nonprocessed food, that message is aimed at a pretty elite demographic. The average household eats fast food. On every interstate highway exit from coast to coast, do you see clusters of farmer's markets and veggie stands or rows of fast-food franchises?

And the truth is that we're more than a nation in a hurry: We're a nation of people who do not like to be told what to eat and when to eat it. And when it comes to nutrition, trust me: The City Gym Boys are speaking your language. Would I prefer to be eating fresh sea bass every day? Well, it sounds good—but I can't afford it. Most of us can't afford it.

So, as a result, we do what you should be doing, too: After we eat at McDonald's, we simply make sure to exercise to burn off the calories.

Here's a great example for us all: As I'm writing this, Michelle Obama has taken a little criticism for having a fast-food lunch of a burger, fries and a shake. Was her meal sensible? Of course it was! This is a woman who obviously does her gym time. This is a woman who clearly has things in balance. She didn't get those arms from sitting around idly.

I guarantee you that Michelle Obama worked off those calories. It's pretty inspiring to see a fitness role model in the White House— a woman who walks the walk as much as she talks the talk. She obviously keeps her kids physically active as well. This is a woman who is leading as a parent as well as a first lady.

When we got off the plane and arrived at our hotel in New Orleans, the first thing we did was go to the hotel gym. And working out in the hotel gym is exactly what we did. Within forty minutes to an hour, those calories had been deleted.

That night, the scene repeated itself, in a way, at a cocktail reception. As usual, even though we were dressed a little more stylishly for the high-profile bash, we were getting all sorts of attention (people see the muscles and do double takes, even when the muscles are masked by shirts or jackets). Anyway, we head for the bar and the bartenders give us a weird look as if to say, "You guys actually drink? And you want something other than a light beer?"

Why shouldn't we? We work out, so it's not a problem to enjoy a drink. Although I'm not a big drinker, I still enjoy a vodka and cranberry juice once in a while. The key is to burn off the calories that you take in.

Life is all about moderation; fitness isn't an all-or-nothing deal. Some people get caught up in a mind-set that's really nothing but an excuse disguised as bad logic. "I can't work out for five days, so what good would two do?" "I can't give up my cocktails, so why work out?" "I could never give up potato chips at lunch, so what's the point of trying to lose weight?" Ridiculous. Yes, when you're working out, you should go all out; remember, work to failure. But how often you do it is your own choice.

Most important, if you see fitness as an all-or-nothing deal, then you're setting yourself up to fail. That kind of thinking starts equating being fit with sacrificing so many of the things you love in life, and like most people, you'll then be less likely to work out. This is

> **"If you see fitness as an all-or-nothing deal, then you're setting yourself up to fail"**

part of the obesity equation, too: With a million diets out there flying at you, hammering you with the gospel that what you eat is why you're fat, how could you *not* believe that getting fit means giving up things you like?

For me feeling fit—not the superficiality of *looking* fit—is such a blessing that walking in the street sometimes I feel almost like, "God, why me? Why am I so lucky? Why am I feeling as if I'm on top of the world?"

But I know the answer. I earned this feeling. I earned the right to rise every day with a smile on my face, knowing I'm being the best I can be. And you'll be there, too—as soon as you stop making food the scapegoat. Or the enemy.

> **"I earned the right to rise every day with a smile on my face"**

We can't say it enough: It's not what you eat, it's what you do. And we're going to keep saying it until someone listens. Of course, in the fitness world, all they say is, "Eat clean, eat clean, eat clean." To many people that message means one thing: calories. But do we know *what* calories? There are good calories. There are bad calories.

On top of which, let's face it: A mom preparing food for her kids has no time or idea how to keep track of which calories are good, and which aren't. She doesn't even have the time when she's shopping after a long day of work to even *count* those calories.

NO, THE REAL PROBLEM is not what you eat—it's the fact that you're not *doing* anything afterward. When was the last time you climbed a few flights of stairs instead of waiting for the elevator? When was the last time you walked to the convenience store instead of drove?

We're not moving our bodies. And regardless of what you're eating (assuming you're not surviving on grubs and roots), if you're not physically active in some way, you will gain weight. Period.

My time in South Africa did more than teach me that happiness doesn't come from material belongings. It was in Cape Town that I first realized how out of touch Americans are with the rest of the world when it comes to food. There's nothing like being around people who don't know where their next meal is coming from to put your perspective on food in the right place.

Focusing all of this energy on what's "good food" and what's "bad food" is not only silly; it's also a waste of energy. Too much unrefined sugar! Too much salt! Not enough protein! Too many carbs! In the meantime, millions of people would give anything to have some or any of that food we discard because we're so obsessed with what we eat.

Think about that for a second: We throw out food while two-thirds of the world eats only for survival. While we pore over the list of ingredients on our breakfast cereal, we're forgetting the most important and basic fact about the things we put in our mouths: In the end—and for the last 50,000 years, ever since we evolved into homo sapiens—food is for energy. Nothing more.

In all the blitz of advertising, in all the media celebration of "foodies" and celebrity chefs, we seem to have forgotten what food is for. Food is not to make us feel good. It has become that. Food is for survival and energy. There are a lot of lands where people remember that, because they don't have the luxury of picking and choosing among designer yogurts.

Have you ever visited a subsistence culture, where one family that grows beans trades them for potatoes at the morning market, and the eel fisherman trades his catch for a bushel of carrots? If you have, you know that food is their fuel—and they have no weight problems.

Desiring food just because you can have it goes against biological nature. But because food has become so huge in the economy—because we're so willing to pay for foods we don't need—food has become crazily overexamined. It was never meant to be the subject of debates. It wasn't meant to be an art form. It wasn't meant, for instance, to spawn the Rudd Center for Food Policy & Obesity at Yale University, where Ivy League brains can gather in a think tank to try to solve obesity by minutely examining our diets—and ignoring our exercise patterns.

There's no Center for Exercise and Fitness Policy at Yale. But there are plenty of universities studying obesity, including the University of Maine, which is looking at twenty schools and 3,000 kids in an ongoing, multiyear research project. Recently, the professor of "exercise science" leading the study concluded that the real problem was "too many calories and too much food, and too much leisure time to eat it."

If I had a Ph.D. in exercise science and I were looking at the data that produced that conclusion, I think I'd conclude that the problem is that *the kids aren't exercising in that leisure time*!

But then, last summer, comes a paper in the prestigious *Journal of the American Medical Association* (*JAMA*) that actually discussed the possibility of taking obese children away from their parents because poor parenting has promoted obesity. And check out the first reasons cited for childhood obesity: junk food in the house and "lack of opportunity for physically active recreation."

Wait. One study says children have too much time to eat. Another suggests a scary and radical solution, because the kids don't have the "opportunity" to exercise. What am I supposed to believe?

That's easy: If kids are active—the way kids used to be active—they are not going to be obese. So why didn't the *JAMA* authors suggest getting the kids and parents to work out together? Was that too radical a thought? It seems that in their eyes, it would be easier to break up families than to recommend curing the plague from the bottom up. This kind of thinking—by some of our smartest people, mind you—is the result of treating food not as fuel but as some sort of magic bullet.

The bottom line is that we're lazy, because we're allowed to be, and so we simply expect the food to do the work. We tell ourselves, "If I go with a light beer and low-sodium crackers, I'll lose weight." Think about that for a moment. If you're not exercising, how in the world is a "light" beer going to help your health?

Of course, trying to overcome the advertising and marketing arms of the food companies is always going to be an uphill battle. They're always looking for a way to make you feel as if what you eat is the key to your well-being, all the while packing their products in new "family size" boxes. (Have the families gotten bigger, or the people in them?)

But face it: We're going to keep eating snacks whether they're low-fat, high-fat, no-salt or tons-of-salt. We are a nation of quick-fix, quick-satisfaction individuals. America's diet is not going to change significantly, no matter how many times you hear that the trend is to eat healthier. When was the last time you saw a fast-food franchise that touted tofu?

We have to be realistic. The reason we're failing on the nutrition side, no matter how much research is done, is that we're not using any kind of self-control, or internal logic.

We listen to government nutritionists and doctors tell us what to eat on a daily basis—and that's just not realistic. In fact, it does more harm than good. It works against the goal. The so-called "good food" mentality puts the compulsive eaters in the exact place they want to be.

Compulsive eaters are consumed by food, and then they go out and eat, without exercising. Until we take the focus away from food and eating and put the excitement back in physical activity, nothing is going to change. The truth is that some people simply don't like to be told not to do things. The moment you tell them not to eat something, they *want* to eat it.

So the key is discipline. If we know a food has more palm oil in it than it should, the answer isn't to switch to the snack with canola or grape seed oil that doesn't taste as good; the answer is to simply not eat as much. Besides, what happens when you switch to a "healthier" snack? You eat more of it.

Having a pack of Hostess Twinkies every day for a month is going to send my cholesterol into the stratosphere. But one pack every two months isn't going to make any difference to *any* part of my body. A

brisk mile walk to a farmer's market, an amazing homemade chocolate chip cookie from a local baker and a mile walk back home?
That's a recipe for success, and a happy snacker.

Self-discipline is important in every other part of life, isn't it? Aren't
the words "Everything in moderation" great words to live by? But too
often we're thinking, "Everything in the extreme," as in giving up sweets
for a month, then living on chocolate ice cream for the next week.

In New York, great pizza is as much a part of the culture as the
subway system. At a state fair in the Midwest, buttered corn and
fried dough are staples. In the South, fried chicken is part of the
DNA. I ate a lot of fast foods in high school, but I was also extremely active, running track and doing other things to stay fit.

Perhaps you've seen the McDonald's commercial with Dwight
Howard of the Orlando Magic and LeBron James of the Miami
Heat that aired during Super Bowl XLIV in 2010. It features two of
the most talented athletes in the world competing in a one-on-one
slam dunk contest to win a McDonald's value meal. What's most
interesting about the commercial to me is not that they're competing for a Big Mac and fries but that they spend the majority of the
commercial participating in physical activity. Running, jumping and
eventually shattering a backboard, the two athletes are the embodi-
ment of "It's not what you eat, it's what you do."

Granted, this is a commercial that they were both paid to do,
but it's not hard to believe that both Dwight and LeBron enjoy fast
food in real life. Fast food is hardly the only thing in their diet, but
because they train so hard, they know that they can eat whatever
they want in moderation. These men are paid to keep their bodies in
top shape—it's their job. But even for those of us who aren't professional athletes, being fit and living a healthy life is just as rewarding
as it is for LeBron.

BUT LET'S TAKE A LOOK at food and its rightful role in our lives
from a different angle. Let's examine cultures. I'm from a Carib-

bean culture. My parents, grandparents, aunts and uncles grew up eating what American nutritionists would call "bad food." They are not obese. They do not have a weight issue. In Jamaica and Cuba, people are naturally active. They walk, they run and they move.

And while we're talking about cultures, try telling the people of Italy not to eat big meals or their bread, pasta, cheese and salami. They are not a fat culture. In fact, they have admirably low obesity rates.

Of course, Italians offset their eating with lots of daily physical activity. They walk the streets of mountain villages, traveling by foot on farmland roads to get to the village in the first place. They ride bikes on a continent that long ago understood that bicycling is a real and necessary way of getting around. They don't choose escalators and elevators over footpaths and sidewalks.

"The key is discipline"

The reality is that in most cultures, what we call "bad food" is part of their traditional cuisine—but they are active enough to compensate. But we aren't; we always want an excuse, and we always want a way out. If we blame food and diet, we can ignore our laziness. If we don't acknowledge that the cause of obesity is inactivity, then we don't have to look ourselves in the mirror and ask, "Why aren't you walking to work instead of driving? Why aren't you walking down the hill to the grocery store?"

And why aren't you doing simple body weight exercises in your living room?

Eat and drink the things that make you happy in life. If you can be productive, healthy and happy while eating and drinking the foods you like—in moderation—then that's the way to go. Obsessing about whether they're good foods or bad foods; fretting over their potential to help or harm you; denying yourself their even occasional pleasure; poring over calorie counts—not only is all of this largely pointless, it does something even worse. It ruins food's ability to enhance your life. Hey, just because food is primarily fuel doesn't mean you can't enjoy it.

Speaking of "good" and "bad," let's talk about alcohol. Alcohol would fall under the "bad drink" category, right? But it isn't "bad," any more than a fast-food cheeseburger is a "bad food." When it comes to drinking, alcohol consumption is no different than the "good food, bad food" consumption argument: It's a misguided debate. Have the glass of red wine. (It's good for your heart.)

Now, if you're drinking hard liquor so often that the calories are piling up, in the long run your problem isn't going to be the calories; it's going to be your liver. But if you like to have a drink or two, have them and then make sure that the next day you burn the calories.

Don't deprive yourself of the glass or two of wine, or the cocktail after a stressful day, because you mistakenly think that what you put in your body determines health, weight or happiness. Moderation and discipline are still the keys.

But if we're talking beer, be careful not to fall into the modern traps of the "light" beers trend. It's widely accepted in the beverage industry that "light" drinkers are far more likely to drink a significantly larger amount of beer—even though the difference between regular and light beer is just a one-sixth drop in alcohol and calories.

ECONOMICS ALSO PLAYS a role in eating and nutrition decisions, and in low-income neighborhoods, a lot of factors come into play. Let's get real: There's no Whole Foods in the Bronx or South Central or Roxbury. And even if there were, why would a single mother of three kids, working two jobs to support her family, buy a four-dollar bottle of organic apple juice or a two-dollar bag of apple chips when she can get a dollar cheeseburger and a two-dollar bottle of soda?

In 2010, the single best-selling product in American grocery stores was carbonated beverages, and baked desserts, pizza, and sodas were the top three sources of calories for American children.

Sure, in an ideal world we would all be able to have the best food—the best cuts of meat, the cereals stocked with grains and lately, the vegetables grown in our own gardens. (The "locavore" movement is fabulous—for people who have the time, and yard space, to cultivate their own garden!) It's encouraging that we're going organic with our food and biodynamic with our beverages, but how many Americans can actually afford this stuff?

The most troublesome thing about this new wave of urging "good" food on us is that it seems in so many ways to punish the poor. If you can't buy mesclun salad for your kids, you're made to feel as if you're not a good parent.

And let's face it: The kids who crowd the corner stores after school lets out every day at 3:00 p.m. make it pretty obvious that no matter what they eat in school, they're going to fill up on sweets and junk. I know about the corner store from experience. I was in that corner store with that little daily allowance every day, and all I wanted was candy. I didn't want to buy food. I wanted to buy the candy laid out in the window. I had the menu in my head. Nothing was going to stop me.

But nothing ever stopped the joy I got from running track and playing sports, either.

Parents can't legislate the snack syndrome. They can try—as some parents in North Philadelphia did last spring, when they crowded around a corner store, in safety vests and walkie-talkies, to keep kids from buying snacks before school last spring. Was it fair to the shop owner? No. Was it fair to the kids? Of course not.

Those parents could have spent their energy much more effectively by taking a long walk with their children after school and working out with them—spending some quality time teaching them body weight exercises.

Meanwhile, last March a sales director for a store in Philadelphia bought $500 worth of apple chips that cost 15 cents a bag . . . and had to throw them out because no one bought them.

Kids and their need for sugar is a relationship we're never going to break up. I had to laugh last summer when I read about a five-year-old boy in El Paso who'd stolen his mother's minivan and driven it into a pole. The officers asked the little boy where he was going.

"To buy candy," said the kid.

We pride ourselves on being a nation of leaders. We pride ourselves on being a nation that leads. Well, it's time to lead by activity. It's time to take action—literally. It's time to wake up to the simplest of facts: It's not what you eat, it's what you do.

STILL NOT CONVINCED? Well, here's another way of looking at the food-versus-movement question: You can't look at people and tell what food they eat, can you? No matter what their size, you have no idea what kind of diet they have. A thin guy might be eating candy bars. A fat person might be on an Atkins diet. You don't know if either one consumed 1,000 or 5,000 calories that day.

But you can make *this* judgment and know that you're probably right: If a person is fit, that person is most likely an active person. And if a person is overweight, he or she is most likely not active enough, thus not burning enough calories. Period.

Let's not ignore the obvious correlation between working out and food habits, as anyone who works out regularly knows. When you're being physically active and your focus is on exercising, you tend not to think so much about food. But when you're not active, your sole focus is on food. If you're not active, you're going to be more stressed, and the more stressed you are, the more likely you'll be to reach for the cookies. As a nation, if we emphasize activity, food falls into its natural place: as an energy source, as a pleasure.

We respond to rewards. If you start being active and you see good results from your hard work, you're less likely to consume as much because you don't want to slow down your progress. You're training hard, and your friends and loved ones can see the results. Why mess it up?

That feeling of getting better, stronger and more confident is contagious. There's so much satisfaction to be gained from taking your life into your own hands and legs and shoulders. With every rep, you're taking *action*.

> **If a person is fit, that person is most likely an active person**

Whether it's doing those 200 sit-ups on a personal challenge and collapsing in happiness at the end, or choosing to walk thirty blocks instead of taking the subway; whether it's reaching that hundredth push-up or completing eight laps around the local high school's track; whether it's finally being able to hold your own in an intense hour of pick-up basketball at the gym or power walking a mile through your neighborhood at dawn with your best friend—it doesn't matter how you get your workout in. It's not only physically rewarding, it's psychologically powerful. A great workout is a natural high.

IN CONCLUSION, IT'S SIMPLE: Calories in, energy out. If there's a deficit, you lose weight. If there's a surplus, you gain. Most fitness experts will agree on that.

How you get there will always be subjective. High protein? More carbs? Less fat? Less salt? We'll argue about that stuff until kingdom come. But at the end of the day, people don't like to be told what to do, and for change to truly take place, it has to come from you alone—achieving it *your* way.

But there's one sure way to get you to control your body's future: Channel your self-discipline into moving your body and forget about using it to eat the "right" foods. It's time to abandon the talking and theorizing and get on with the business of moving our bodies. You've taken your own first step toward change by picking up this book. Now it's time to take your destiny into your own hands.

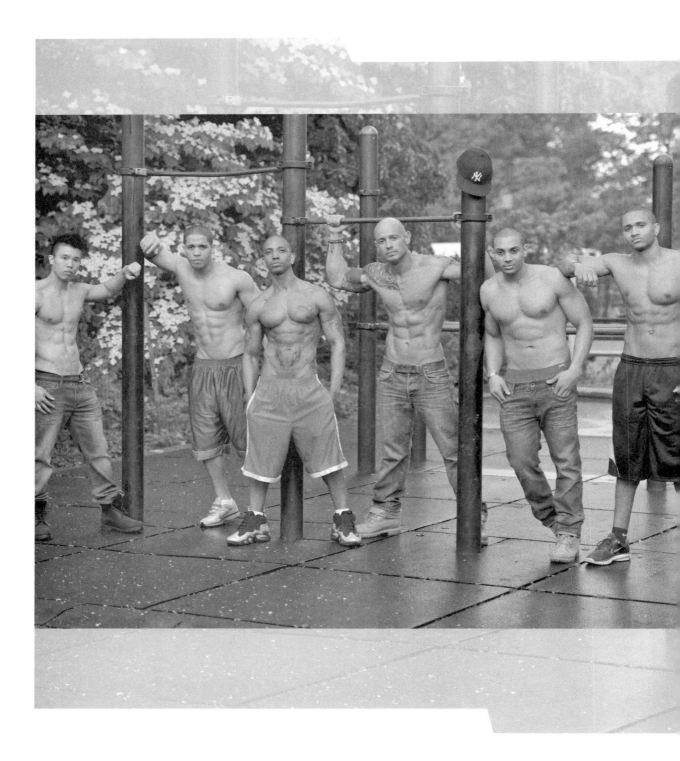

CHAPTER 5

NATURAL IS THE ONLY OPTION

THE CITY GYM BOYS ARE KNOWN FOR APPEARING AT parades and festivals across New York City—from the Puerto Rican Day Parade on Fifth Avenue, to the Brazilian Day Festival, to the African-American Day Parade in Harlem. The fun starts when we get off the subway, carrying our backpacks, and find a quiet side street and start stripping down, looking to get that quick pump. People start walking by, doing double takes, totally confused: Who are those guys?

We were Clark Kents on the subway. We're about to turn into Supermen.

Now, on the sidewalk, everyone gets into their own zone. We've got our music on in our headphones, and we start doing what we each have to do to get a nice pump, get the blood flowing. We start working out. Some of us are doing pull-ups on scaffolding. Some of us are doing push-ups on the sidewalk. It's like getting ready for the Super Bowl. It's physical, and it's mental. You can feel the adrenaline.

Then, finally, we take off the shirts and rub on the cocoa-butter cream, and by that time people are gathering around, going crazy.

These parades and festivals go on for hours and hours. We know from the moment we take the shirts off that we won't have a moment to ourselves until we put our shirts back on. There'll be packs of girls, and boys, people of all ages, following after us, whistling, cheering, amazed. At the Brazilian Day Festival, people are wondering, "Are they Brazilian?" At the Colombian Independence Day Festival, they're saying, "Are they Colombian?" The truth is, demographically and ethnically, our group consists of a little bit of everyone.

But the whole group doesn't get to crash the festivals or do the modeling gigs or work at the schools. Not all of the guys who approach us to be part of the group understand what it takes to be a City Gym Boy. There's the looks, of course. But there's a lot more: the physical and mental dedication. The passion for community service. The weekly commitment to volunteering at the Boys & Girls Club of Harlem.

And, of course, no drugs. I interviewed a guy from the gym recently, a guy I've known a long time. He wanted to be in the group. But I saw that his body had changed—likely due to steroids. I said to him, "You know, our guys have to be clean. And it's better if you let me know, 'cause you can stop."

So he confessed: He'd done a photo shoot and admitted to doing a cycle of testosterone. "Just once," he said. "To make me feel better emotionally."

I couldn't let him join the team. It's difficult to turn down a friend. But if you're using, I'll tell you right at the start that this is not acceptable within the City Gym Boys. Our goal is to train hard

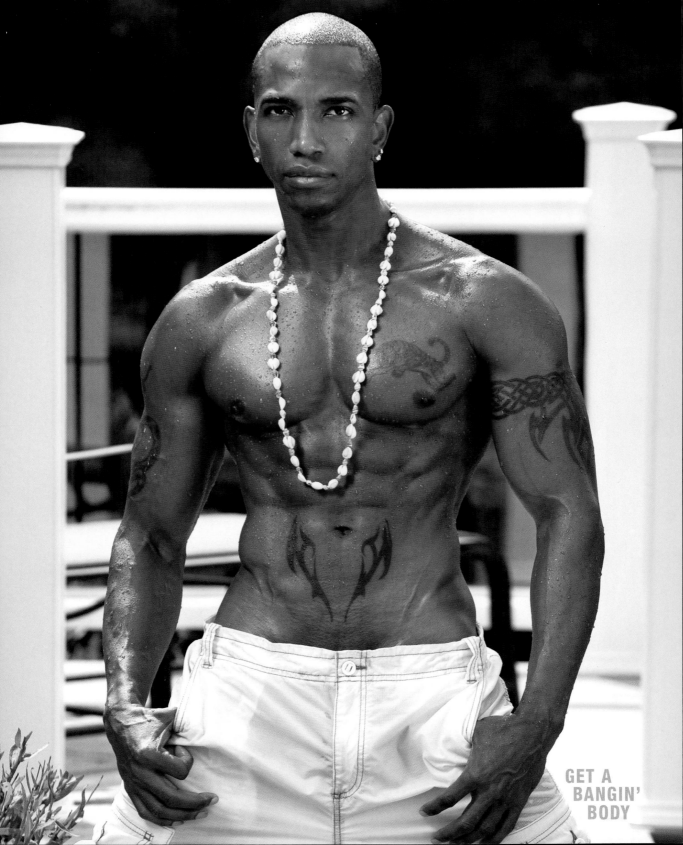

GET A
BANGIN'
BODY

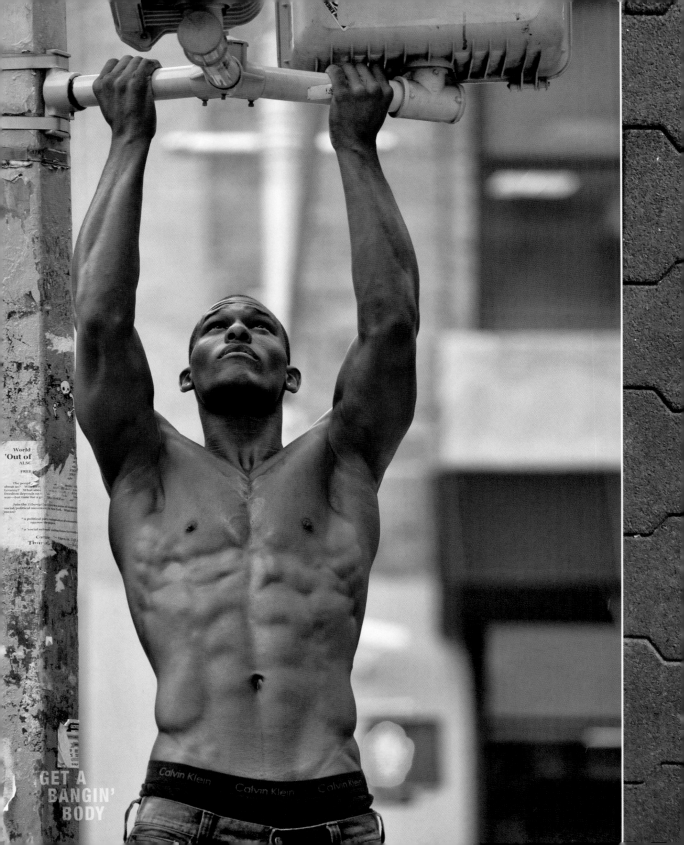

GET A
BANGIN'
BODY

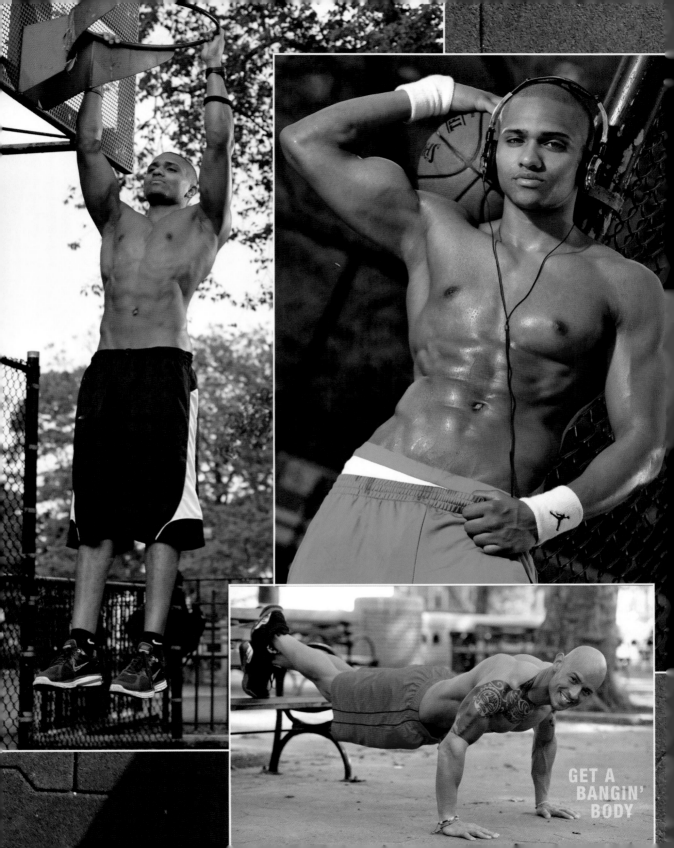

GET A
BANGIN'
BODY

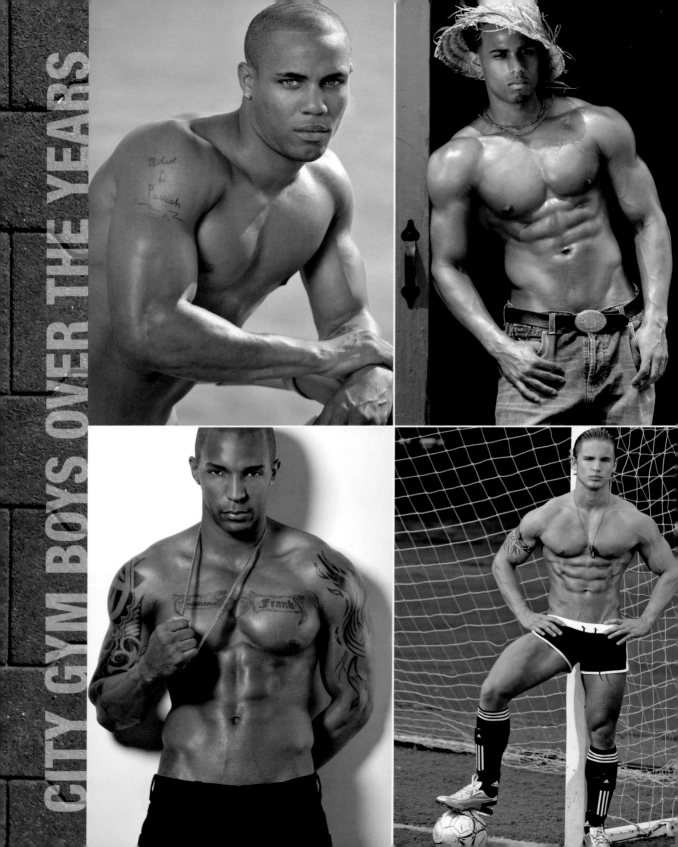

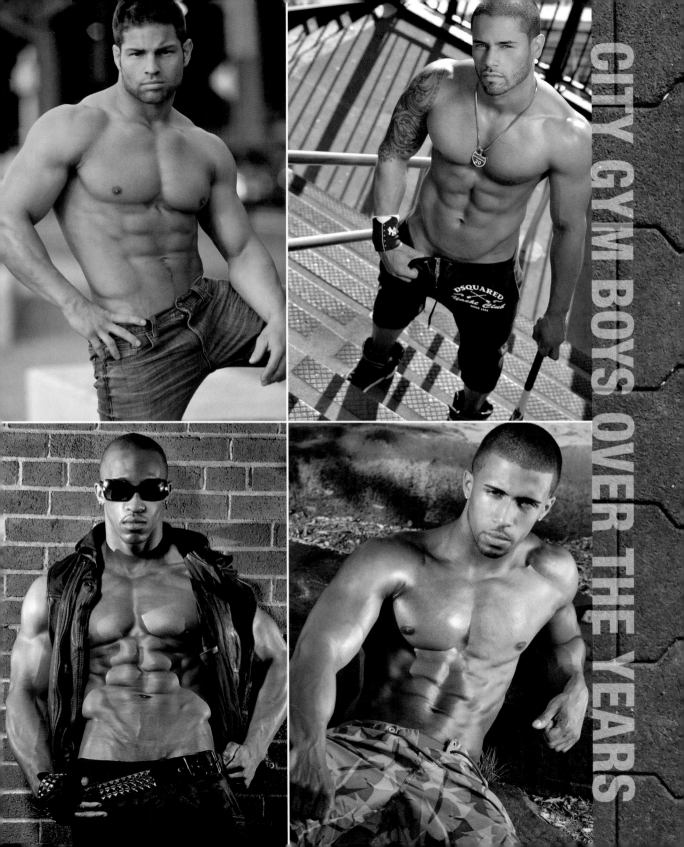

CITY GYM BOYS OVER THE YEARS

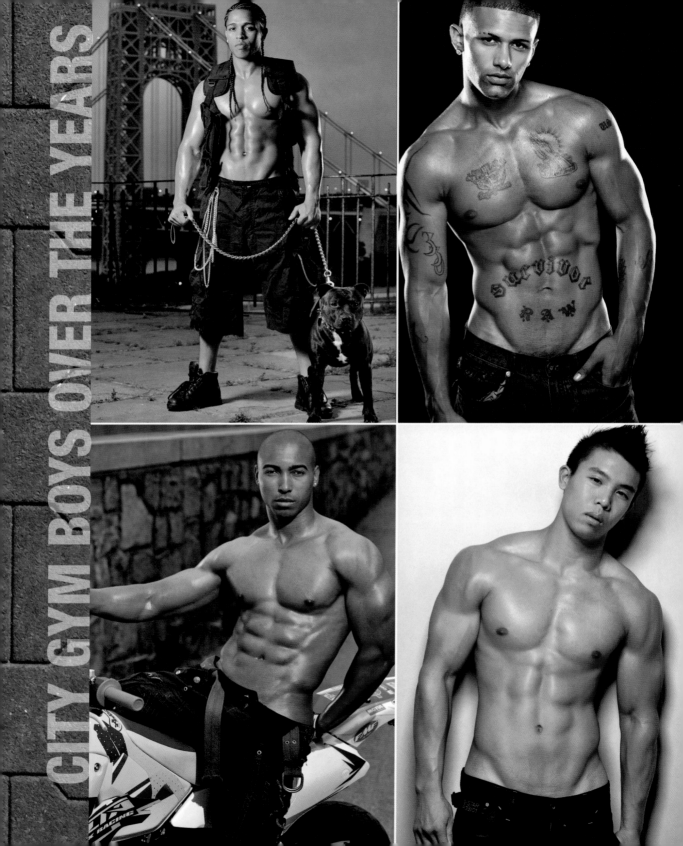

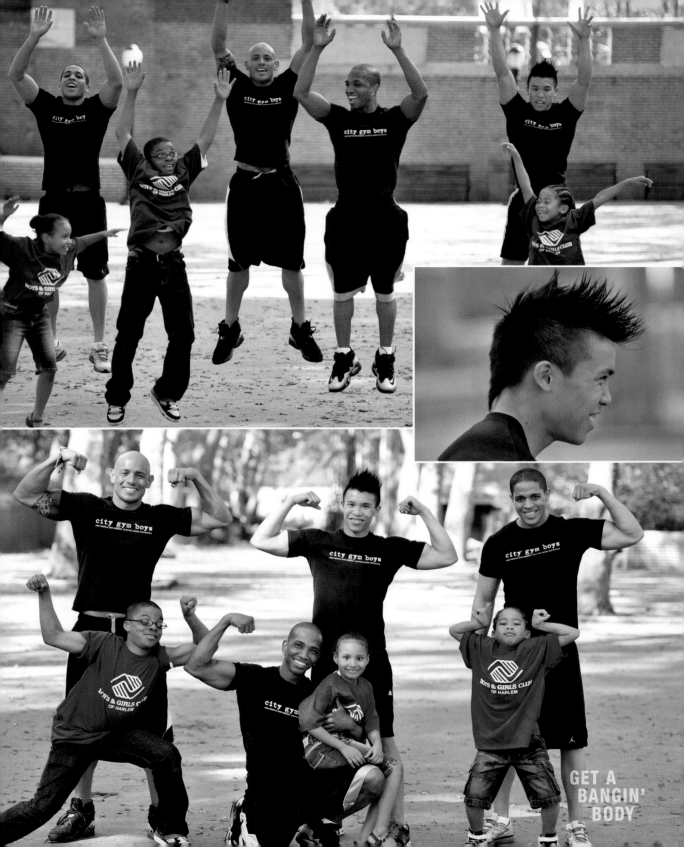

GET A BANGIN' BODY

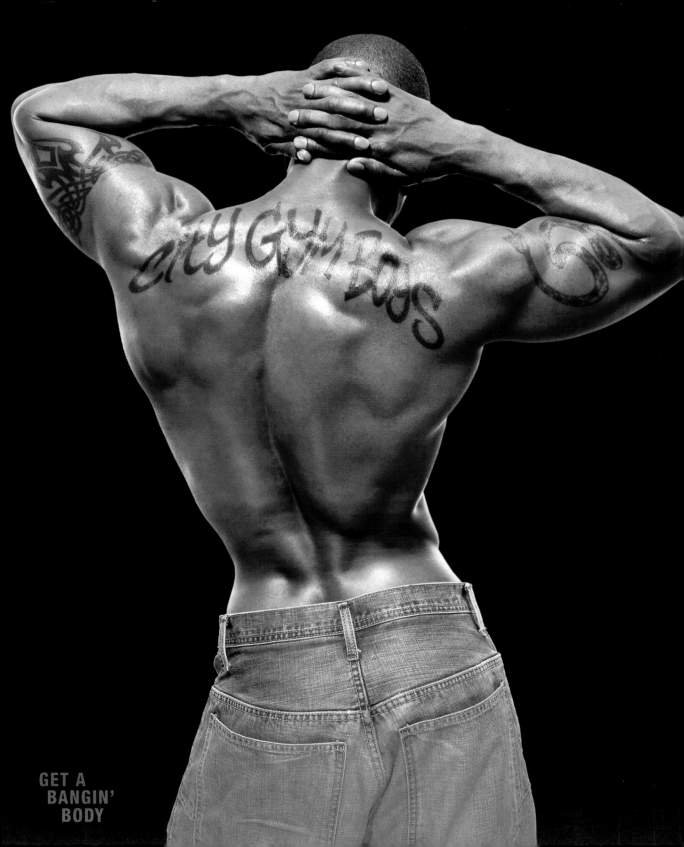

GET A
BANGIN'
BODY

in the gym and create a bangin' physique the old-fashioned, natural way. We're not about fleeting overnight success—we're about hard work.

You don't want to be strolling along 135th Street during the Harlem Week festival, basking in your moment of glory, knowing that you use enhancement drugs. You'd be cheating not only yourself but also all of those people in the 'hood who are looking to you for inspiration.

When I was competing in bodybuilding, I felt the pressure from a lot of people to get big quicker. I never gave into that. I never felt that I would be me if I used enhancement to win. It wasn't a question of the potential guilt. I just never felt like I needed to do anything unnatural. I said no to it then, and I say no to it now.

Steroids are always an option in my world, but for me and the City Gym Boys it isn't.

Truth is, I have never done any kind of drug in my life. I'm not into experimenting. Never smoked a joint, never done a line of coke—that's just not the kind of person I am. I was never the person to say, "I'll try it." I was always the one to say, "I don't think so." And that feeling just gained momentum. It was like working out: The more I kept saying no, the more I knew I would always say no.

When I was younger, it was coming at me so much that I found that the more I said no, the more I was proving to myself that I was a strong person. The fact that I was doing so well in the competitions helped, too. I was not getting first place against drug users, but I would get second or third. I felt that if I was beating a lot of the guys who were juiced, even if I didn't get the top prize, in my world I'm really winning because I'm 100 percent natural.

Medically, it's been proven: The path of steroids is a risky one. The younger City Gym Boys are already trained to go natural, because the public schools have wisely started to preach against the drugs in health classes.

The natural path to fitness is the road to take. And if you have any doubt, all you have to do is look at the faces of the people who approach us at the festivals. They see bodies that are perfectly pro-portioned, not ballooned and grotesque. They see smooth skin, not acne pockmarks. Their admiration is a whole lot more satisfying than a trophy. It's the most incredible feeling when we turn a corner and start to walk through a crowd, and people's eyes make their way toward us.

But the funny thing is, after awhile it's not so much about ego anymore. It's more like, "I have to continue this"—for them, not for myself. You're changing peoples' lives. After all the time in the gym, when you actually take it out there onto the street and realize how impressive and inspiring you are to others, that's when it becomes clear that you can't stop. You have a mission: to get as many people as possible to want to follow your path.

And so you'll be going back to the gym. It becomes a cycle, a cycle of work and pleasure. More time in the gym means a more effective show at the parades and festivals, where people keep coming up and saying things like, "I love what you're doing," and, "I guess I have to join a gym." And even if they're saying that jok-ingly, you can tell that you've already made a difference—especially when they approach you thinking you must be doing some amazing, unreal workout, and you tell them that they can start changing their own lives with a few simple body weight workouts and a new com-mitment to *activity*.

It's hard for anybody to see a group of attractive cut guys walk-ing down the street, with crowds of men and women drawn like fil-ings to a magnet, and not be reminded that maybe they themselves ought to be spending five or ten minutes a day on a treadmill. When you're not at your own best and you see six guys with six-packs who are where you'd want to be in your fantasy, it gives you motivation to achieve your fitness goals.

I'm here to tell you that your body can be anything you want it to be, and when your body is at its peak, your brain benefits, too.

> "**Your body can be anything you want it to be**"

SPEAKING OF "BRAINS," I met Jelani at a festival in Harlem. He's a sophomore at Williams College and a graduate of the Ethical Culture Fieldston School—one of the most prestigious prep schools, with more famous alumni than you can count (including *New York Times* executive editor Jill Abramson and John Lennon's son Sean).

When he's not in school, you'll usually find him by my side in one of our middle-of-the-night workouts at J's Big Gym in Washington Heights, surrounded by guys who might have never finished high school, or who might be finishing up a tough day at the brokerage. The late-night gym community isn't concerned with where you're from or how much you make. It's a sanctuary for those who want to work hard and shape their body.

This is a young guy with his eye on the prize. I have a feeling that Jelani might be the next name on that boldfaced Fieldston alumni list.

JELANI MEDFORD

I'm probably the only City Gym Boy who spends the majority of his year in a college quad surrounded by the green hills of northwestern Massachusetts. I'm also probably the only Williams College student with a tribal tattoo of a wolf on his shoulder—a representation of my love and respect for animals. I also have another tattoo on my chest. It reads, "I can be anything I want to be, as long as I am The Best."

It's a philosophy that my dad instilled in me at a very young age: Always give your all and be the best that you can be in anything that you put your mind to. That's exactly what I plan to do. I think I fit well in my roles of being both a Williams student and a City Gym Boy. Achieving a degree in psychology is one of my most recent personal goals, and I plan to achieve it.

There are about 2,000 students here at Williams, and there's nothing but miles of green countryside in every direction. You could argue that Williams (located in Williamstown, Massachusetts) is in the middle of nowhere, but that's one of the great things I like about being here: that there are so few distractions. I love the contrast with New York. Williamstown is a small town with a great community, and I love it up here. Of course, I love Harlem, too, which is where I grew up and first met Charles.

It was one day during Harlem Week, the festival in mid-August where the whole neighborhood hits the streets to network, showcase products and talents, and support our community.

That day, I happened to be wearing a tank top. I'd come a long way from that skinny, scrawny kid who was ashamed to take his shirt off. Whether I was at the beach or in the park, I was always self-conscious. I come from a household where fitness was always a priority and both of my parents have always been in great shape. My mom was a trophy-winning bodybuilder and continues her career as a personal trainer. My dad is an ex-Marine who continues to stay in shape through running, weight training and basketball.

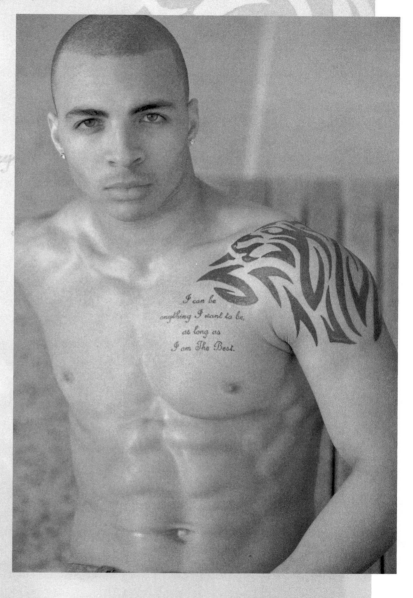

As a son of two highly active parents, I've always been active myself: Football, basketball, salsa dancing and capoeira (the Brazilian art form that combines dance and martial arts) are some of the ways I like to keep my body moving. I even picked up hockey after I took a job at the skating rink at Chelsea Piers in New York a few years ago.

But the summer after I graduated from eighth grade at The Cathedral School, I went up to Rochester to help my uncle who was doing construction and renovation, and everything changed. When I wasn't painting or up on a roof, there wasn't really much to do. My uncle had a home gym, so I began to work out when I wasn't working for him. I figured it would help me as a freshman trying out for the football team at Fieldston.

But soon I began to really enjoy the routine. I was immediately addicted. I hadn't really noticed how much of a difference the summer workouts had made to my physique until I came home to the city later that summer and everyone commented on my transformation. My mom said, "Whoa, what happened to you?" My friends saw me and were inspired to start working out themselves.

This all did a lot for my self-esteem. I started feeling more comfortable speaking to people and asserting myself. When you're in great shape, and people notice, all sorts of things happen: Your posture is better. Your attitude is better. Your confidence is better. Walking into a room with strangers, you feel confident about yourself. In fact, the confidence and self-esteem I developed through changing my body probably had a lot to do with me getting into one of the most prestigious colleges in the country.

ON THAT DAY during Harlem Week, I was proud of the way I looked. When I first met Charles, he explained the idea behind the group. I remembered seeing him and the other City Gym Boys earlier that day walking proudly through the streets, stopping to take pictures and promote their calendar. I knew that I had a CGB body, but it was hidden beneath my tank top. It wasn't until, encouraged by Charles, I decided to join in on one of the pictures and flash my abs that I realized my own City Gym Boy potential.

That sparked the beginning of my City Gym Boy career, and I've been on board ever since. I knew there was something unique about the City Gym Boys. I was joining not just an organization but a brotherhood—guys of all different cultures and backgrounds, who shared a passion for motivating and inspiring others to take ownership of their physique.

Just as cool was the fact that I'd found a guy with whom I could work out with any time, day or night. Sometimes, a workout at 11:00 p.m. is the best workout you can have. It's the perfect way to end a day. No matter what happened during the day, good or bad, you can put it all behind you. And I always do.

Granted, there are a lot of ways to unwind from a stressful day—like drugs or alcohol. But for me, that's never going to be an option. I don't drink or smoke—never have, never will. But a late-night workout at the gym with Charles by my side sets me up for a great next day. Exercise is almost like a vacation, an escape. Something about working out frees your mind; you're exerting all of this mental and physical force into this amazing workout, and if it's the last thing you do during the day, it almost guarantees that tomorrow's going to go well. Sure, I might be sore, fatigued or tired the next day. But it's great for my studies, because it keeps my head clear and it helps with time management.

With my commitment to working out consistently, excelling in my studies and being an active member of the Williams community, I don't have time to procrastinate and push things off until later. I feel like I get my work done best when there's pressure on me. For me, there's no time to dillydally.

And no, I've never done steroids and never will. I was never tempted. In middle school and high school we had health classes, and the dangers of drugs, particularly steroids, were always the main focus. I never wanted to abuse my body in any way. I'm going to focus on my work ethic and achieve my goals the way they were meant to be achieved—the clean, natural way.

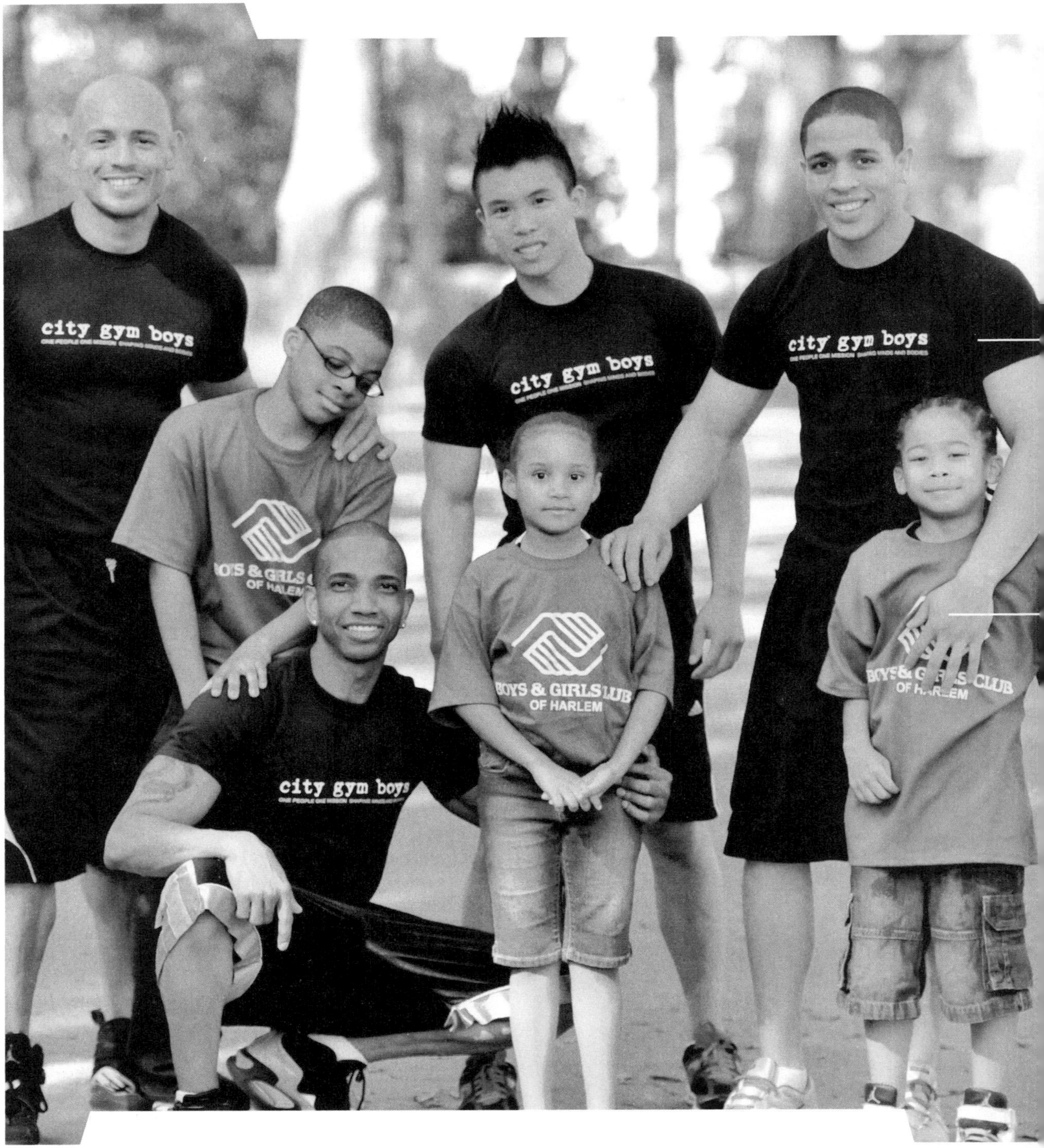
city gym boys
city gym boys
city gym boys
city gym boys
BOYS & GIRLS CLUB
OF HARLEM

FIND YOUR MOTIVATION, MIND YOUR INTENSITY

IT'S PUT-UP OR SHUT-UP TIME. ALTHOUGH YOU HAVEN'T seen a gym since the Clinton administration, and the only exercise you get is (sometimes) climbing the stairs, you've vowed to give it your all. You're not embarking on this course because your wife said you should or your kids got on your case or because your coworkers have been teasing you. This time it's real, because like anything in life that really matters, the only person who can persuade you to take the first step is you. And now you've made the vow.

Okay, let's stop right here. Before you simply step into sweats and start your first push-ups in the basement, know this: The first step is not physical. The first step is *all mental*. So, first things first: Get your head in the right place.

Let's start with your attitude toward your workout.

THE FIRST STEP IS being aware that you have to give every rep the effort it deserves. Effort is everything. You have to push your body to its limit on every rep of every set that you do. I repeat: *every rep of every set you do*. You don't expect a bank account with a few dollars in it to grow to a million, right? Then you can't expect to change your life with a half-baked effort in your exercises.

Now, everyone's maximum effort is different. You'll think you know your limit, but you probably don't. You can push harder than you think you can. You're not going to kill yourself. A lot of people are afraid of working hard, and if you're one of those people, push that fear aside. You *have* to push yourself. You're using your own guidelines to push your own body. With that effort, you'll get to today's limit.

Maybe you might simply try *walking* today—as long and fast as you can—instead of running. Tomorrow you can increase the pace and distance. But keep in mind: You cannot level out, no matter if you're a beginner or a City Gym Boy. The fitter you are, the harder you have to try. The body is constantly changing, and if you're not getting better, you're getting worse.

The important thing is to max out, whether that max is two hundred sit-ups, or two. If you're going to do five sets of ten push-ups, max out on that first set. Take a quick break, get the heart rate down, then go back and max out on second set, and make the last set the best.

In other words, *work to failure*. These are powerful words, and they're essential if you're going to keep your new vow. Working out isn't doing all that it can do if you walk away without feeling drained, tested and exhausted. Working to failure every time is the key to changing your body. If you're not working to failure, in every workout, you're not giving your body the best effort. If you set a goal of doing fifty push-ups, and upon reaching fifty you know you can do more but you stop, you're not giving your body the best effort. If you're sprinting at the end of your two-mile loop through the neighborhood and you've got more gas in the tank, but decide to wind down, you're not giving your body the best effort. None of the physical improvements you're hoping for is going to happen if you don't push—then shatter—the envelope.

Trust me: You'd be surprised, if not amazed, at how far you can push your body right now. Today. At this very moment. You want that body now, don't you? So why wouldn't you start your hardest right now? Push yourself like a champion until you've worked to failure, *starting right now.*

Some people are religious about going to the gym but still aren't seeing results. If you're like that, my guess is that you're going in with the wrong attitude—which is easy to do. A lot of gyms are laid out like indoor country clubs to draw high-rolling clients looking for a status membership. They offer distractions by the dozens. Watching the financial news while you're on the treadmill, checking out the ladies, thinking about the banana/yogurt shake out in the lounge—these aren't prime motivators for a bangin' body. But don't blame the gyms.

"But I get bored!" You do? That means you're not challenging yourself. If you're really challenging yourself, intensity, commitment and focus make boredom impossible.

You want to socialize? Fine. But don't expect to see results. And the next time you feel bored when you're working out, know that you're not really working out hard.

The next time you work out ask yourself, "Am I working out even close to my potential? Even close to my max?" If your answer is no, you should adopt this line of thinking: Workout time is *me* time. I'm doing this to take care of *me*.

And the great thing about body weight workouts is all you have

> **"The first step is all mental"**

to do is find a place where it's just you and your body—a park, an empty school field, your office—and focus is on nothing but the bangin' body you'll build. But no matter where you choose to exercise, one question remains the same: How are you going to be able to make yourself commit?

And the answer is by finding true motivation. For me, that motivation comes from knowing that my physical well-being is as important as my mental state. The two sides *must* be in balance.

We spend so much time planning for the future—school, careers, relationships, retirement—but the future isn't going to mean a thing if our bodies fail. But if we put as much energy into being brilliant and useful physically as we do with our brains, we won't have to worry about the future. More than anything, what has to motivate you is that your future is contingent on you making your body last. You're doing all this work so that your children can have a better life, or so you and your significant other can go off into the sunset hand in hand, but none of that is going to happen if you don't pay attention to that physical package that all of your hopes and dreams depend on.

And speaking of dreams, sleep is such an important part of the formula. Our body changes only in a restful state. If you're up at two in the morning to check the Nikkei stock index in Japan to help give yourself an advantage the next day in the office, just how sound is your judgment going to be on four hours of sleep?

Sure, you've read about those high-powered execs who can get by on four hours of sleep per night. Some people can do that, but most can't. Granted, though, it won't always be possible for us to sleep a sound eight hours. We're busy people. To sleep is like working out: You do the best you can. It's not all or nothing. Get your four or five hours if it's all you can get, but treat your sleep time the way you treat your workout time: Give it what it deserves. Those people who say, "I'll sleep when I'm dead" are kidding themselves.

If you ignore the needs, rhythms and cycles of the body, that brain isn't even going to survive. What good is having a great job, a

> **"The future isn't going to mean a thing if our bodies fail"**

lot of money and a summer house if you've got a big belly, high blood pressure and low energy? That's not healthy living. That's not even living. A heart attack brings all those riches to a new level of meaningless. Until you tell yourself, "This fat around my belly is going to lead to heart disease, high blood pressure and an end to all the good things I'm working like a madman for," you're missing the point. Living for material luxury is a no-win dead end: Get something big, and you're always going to want something bigger, aren't you? But get that feeling that you've accomplished a body that's healthy, and you'll feel satisfaction that no sports car could ever bring you.

I'LL TELL YOU WHO my superhero is when it comes to having balance in life: President Obama. He has a sense of balance between body and mind that every individual should strive for. He is so determined to maintain a balanced life that if he doesn't get his basketball game in or his round of golf or his running, his presidential game is off. I mean, this is a man who decided to remodel the White House tennis court into a basketball court!

You know what's crazy? He's been criticized for playing so much golf—more than either of the Bushes. But what's wrong with walking eighteen holes of golf? That's four miles of walking! And, as we all know, when you're walking, or running, you do some of your best thinking.

Look at the Obamas: He has no stomach, no fat. Mrs. Obama's the same way—and check out those upper arms! If the busiest man in the world can find time to keep moving, what's your excuse? It certainly can't be "I don't have the time."

Looking and feeling good are not superficial things: They reach to your core and make you who you are. How often do you deal with bad news or try to relieve stress by feeling sorry for yourself, drowning those sorrows in beer—and the bad news keeps coming? Did you ever notice how things seem to always be a little better, day in and day out, when you're rising each day healthy and energetic?

I don't have a lot of money. I don't live in the largest apartment. But for me, feeling fit is like being rich. It doesn't matter how much money you have in your pocket; it's how you feel. I feel wealthy and blessed with every step, with every breath, with every walk across the park when I could have taken the bus. I feel wealthy with every run up the stairs when I could have taken the elevator. And you can, too! If your office is on the sixth floor and you don't want to walk up those six flights, take the elevator for three, and then walk the other three. It's little adjustments to your daily routine like this that make all the difference. It doesn't have to be all or nothing. Small steps play a large role in chipping away at the excess pounds.

Set realistic goals for yourself. Maybe you can do only four or five hours a week. That's fine. Two hours a day? Two hours a week? Whatever works.

But keep this in mind: You get out only as much as you put in. You can't expect to get a big paycheck at work if you don't show up and work hard. In the same way, you can't expect to look like a City Gym Boy by working out for just one or two hours a week.

The key is to see yourself in your *own* bangin' body. It's up to you to find your own motivation. You have to find a place in yourself that realizes the importance of working out; a place where the reward far outweighs the sacrifice.

Of course, if you get into a groove and working out becomes the reward in itself, that's even better! But until that happens, you have to find the discipline that will keep you going back, day in and day out. You have to find a place that's going to make you want to make that sacrifice. You don't have to love working out. You don't have to look forward to your workout as the highlight of your day. But you have to know that it's necessary for your physical and mental well-being.

A BIG PART OF the motivation for me is the fact that regardless of my situation before I work out, I know that after I do work out

I'm going to feel better. No matter what position you're in that's taking you in a negative direction—at home, at work, wherever—you're going to feel a whole lot better when you've worked out and you've taken yourself to a place where all the other stuff starts to seem less important.

And don't kid yourself: We may look as if we spend twenty-four hours a day in the gym, but we don't. Even the City Gym Boys have to look for a little extra motivation sometimes. Even me. Sometimes my motivation is to be one of the best bodies of the City Gym Boys—and believe me, that's not easy; these are the best of the best. Sometimes it's just to get rid of some stress. Whatever the case, I know that if I take care of my body, everything else is going to work out.

Envision a picture of where you know you *need* to be: without blood pressure medication. Without so many pounds drooping above your waist. Now envision where, in your fantasies, you *want* to be: where you're catching the eye of that hot lady or good-looking guy. Where you're not afraid to wear that swimsuit at the beach.

Klae Scott, one of our most impressive guys and one of our more amazing athletes, grew up learning how cool it was to have people watch him play on a football field. The last thing he ever thought of was ending up in a City Gym Boys calendar and helping to turn lives around.

Then he learned that although football ends, staying fit is a life-long passion.

"I feel wealthy with every run up the stairs when I could have taken the elevator"

KLAE SCOTT

I was a football player. I wasn't a model. I defined myself by my aggressive style of football. As a high school student in Chicago I was a wide receiver, but when I got to college at the University of Wisconsin–Platteville, they put me on defense. They said they'd never seen a player on offense be so aggressive. So I became a cornerback.

I also became a scholar. One of the great things about Platteville is that every year the grade point average of its student-athletes is higher than its nonathletes. I was using my mind as well as my body, and when I got my bachelor's in business administration, I thought I was headed for the business world.

But I couldn't let football go. So I tried out for the Racine Raiders, a semi-pro team in the Elite Mid-Continental Football League. Don't take that too lightly, either: The Raiders have been around for sixty years and they've put a dozen players in the NFL. And in my rookie year, I not only started but won Defensive Rookie of the Year for the EMCFL.

So when a friend of a friend suggested that I pursue modeling, I said, "I don't model. I don't do that stuff. I play football!" But she was insistent, and she said she had this great photographer. I met him, and he said, "You have a good look. Let's see what we get."

We did some test shots, and the next thing I knew, a booking agent at Ford Modeling Agency saw my pictures and they signed me. Before long, I was doing fashion shows. It was at one of those shows that Epperson, the fashion designer from *Project Runway*, suggested that I get in touch with Charles.

"Have you ever heard of the City Gym Boys?" he asked.

"What are they," I asked. "Dancers?"

He laughed. "Check them out. It's about health and fitness."

I saw the website, saw the calendars, headed to New York, and immediately fell right into their groove. The camaraderie was just great, and the idea of doing something good for the community meant a lot to me. I was always working out anyway, always playing a sport, and people always asked me: "What do you do? What are your workouts?"

So it was an easy transition. And in the past nine years, I've met some pretty amazing people, from Usher to supermodels.

But the most rewarding part of being a City Gym Boy is helping people along their fitness journey and sharing the knowledge of developing a strong body and a strong brain. I don't want to say that I've changed a lot of lives, but . . . well, okay, I *have* changed a lot of lives. That's not bragging. That's just being grateful for the opportunity to convince people of how wonderful it is to stay in shape. There's nothing like bringing someone into the gym and then watching them get hooked.

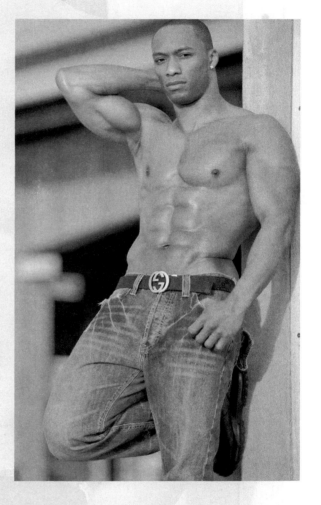

Once they've caught the fitness bug, they don't need me to motivate them. When people say, "You look great!" that's all the motivation they need. Then I tell them, "Guess what? This is just the tip of the iceberg. You can always get better." And the next thing you know, it's their lifestyle. They're helping others, and my work with them is done.

But there's always someone else to teach and convince and recruit. And although my time is limited these days from working two jobs and raising my two-year-old son, Kabel, my work ethic hasn't changed. And it never will.

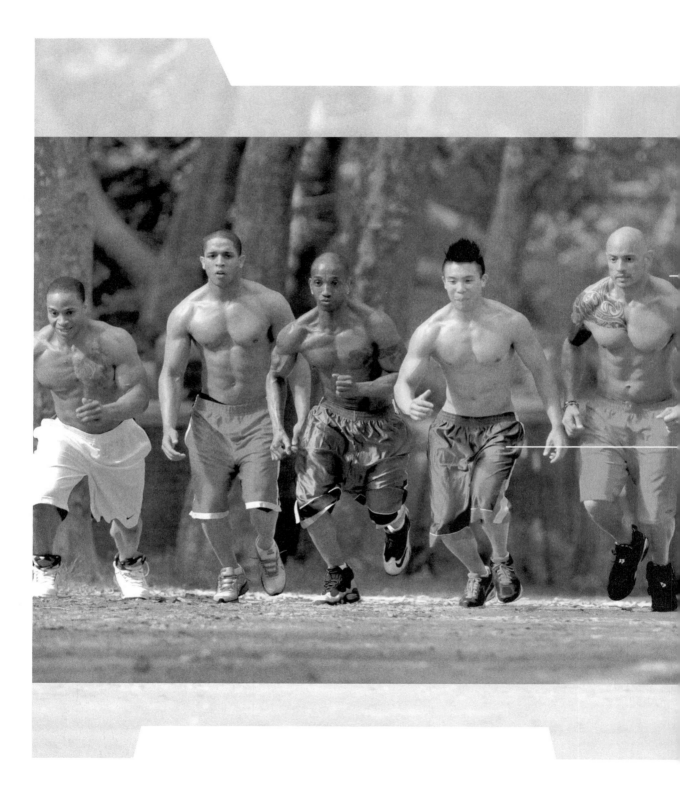

CHAPTER 7

LET'S GET DOWN TO BUSINESS

SOMETIMES I WONDER WHY I'VE BEEN SO LUCKY TO attract so many great people to the City Gym Boys, guys who have great minds and great attitudes and are good citizens. More and more guys from all over want to be a City Gym Boy. Like a lot of coaches, I can be pretty tough. I make a lot of demands on these guys. But they keep coming, and they seem to want to be a part of the positive energy.

I think that may be because I'm a walking example of what I preach: Find the discipline and dedication to change your body, and you'll be amazed at how it will change your life. Your peace of mind, your potential and your ability to do some good in a culture that's never needed it more are all dependent on your being healthy. If you want to make any major contribution to society, you have to be at your best, physically and mentally. And if you are the caretaker for your family, then you must be in your best possible physical shape. Otherwise, you might not be able to help them when they need you most. It's like when, on airplanes, they tell you to put the oxygen mask on yourself first before you help others. You won't be any good to your kids, your friends, your elderly parents or society at large if you're not breathing.

As humans, we all need love; we all need affection. There are certain things you have to have, and the first thing is love. And before you can love others, and get their love in return, you have to love yourself. And the first step toward loving yourself is taking care of yourself, both mind and body. Yes, find the discipline and dedication to change your body and you'll be amazed at how it will change your life.

I'm at the top of my game now, and it's time to spread the word from a position of strength (literally) and experience. And in this book, that's what I've tried to do. But I can take you only so far—the rest is up to you. You owe it not to yourself but to the people around you. Your family, your friends and all your loved ones who are looking to you to lead by example.

Your own bangin' body awaits you. It's time to claim it—starting right now!

" "Before you can love others, and get their love in return, you have to love yourself "

TEN TIPS FOR YOUR BEST WORKOUT

1. FUEL UP:

Try not to eat a meal within three hours of your workout. You will not have the energy to work out if your body is still digesting your most recent meal. It's better to be a little hungry—you'll end up getting a better workout, and you'll burn more body fat.

2. WARM-UP:

Make sure your muscles are warmed up before you start exercising. Do at least ten minutes of cardio activity to get your circulation going. Cold muscles are more likely to get injured.

3. LIMIT REST PERIODS:

Rest periods between sets should be as short as possible—just long enough to bring your heart down a bit and for the muscles to recover. This is not phone time or socializing time. If you're able to maintain an elevated heart rate by keeping your rest periods as brief as possible, your body will go into fat-burning mode while you're also building muscles.

4. KNOW YOUR MUSCLES:

Always be aware of the muscle that you're working when performing an exercise. For example, if you're doing dips, know that you're working your triceps.

5. ISOLATE:

Try to isolate the major muscle that is being worked during the exercise. For example, if you're doing push-ups, make sure your chest is doing most of the work. It's important to connect your brain to the muscle being worked.

6. PRACTICE GOOD FORM:

Good form is *extremely* important for getting good results and avoiding injuries. It requires more focus and energy, but you'll see the results.

7. CONTROL YOUR PACE:

Use a nice, controlled pace—about four seconds each way—for your positive motion (the "hard" part of an exercise) and negative motion (the "easy" part of an exercise). This will allow you to maximize your workout time and will result in much faster and better physical changes.

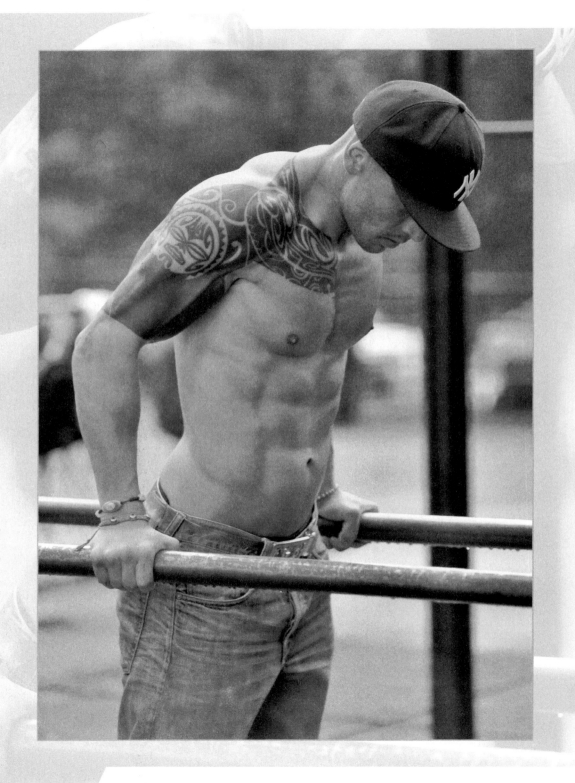

8. EXHALE ON THE HARD, INHALE ON THE EASY:

Exhale on your positive ("hard") motion. This will result in the air filling your lungs naturally as you perform your negative ("easy") motion. Good breathing is as important as good form. Your muscles and brain need oxygen to perform.

9. FEEL THE BURN:

The longer you keep the muscle under stress, the better and faster your body will change. Endure the burn for as long as possible without giving up physically or mentally. Focus on the mental picture of what you want to look like physically, and endure the burn.

10. CHALLENGE YOURSELF:

Your workout should never be easy. Work to muscle failure for every rep of every set, for every workout. Do not hold back for the next set or the next workout! You want that bangin' body today, right? Give your workout all you have today, as if there is no tomorrow.

Note: *Make sure you're healthy enough to work out. As with any new exercise routine, please consult your doctor before beginning this program.*

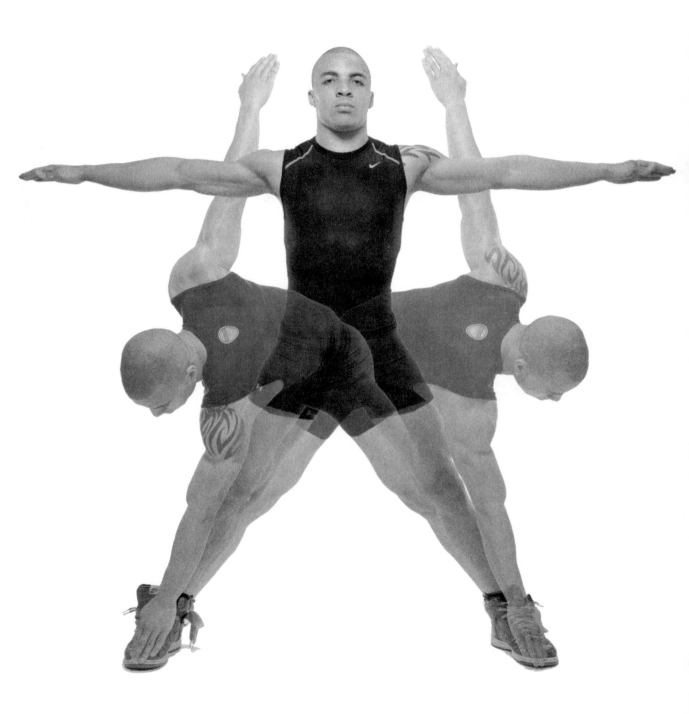

THE
EXERCISES

RUNNING

Keep your knees as high as possible, pumping your arms and running as lightly as possible. Do not put pressure on knees by pounding the floor or ground too hard.

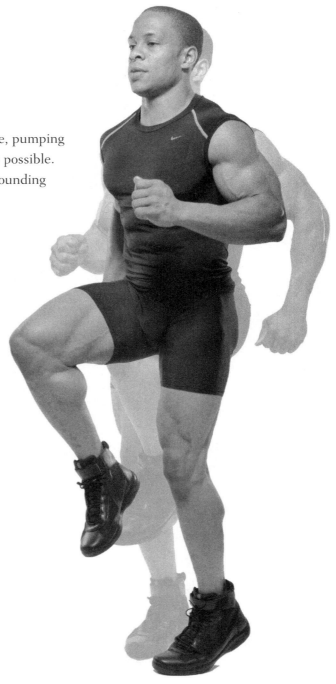

QUICK FEET

Start with your feet slightly wider than your hips, arms out to the side, and lean forward. Move your feet as fast as possible, alternating from one foot to the other.

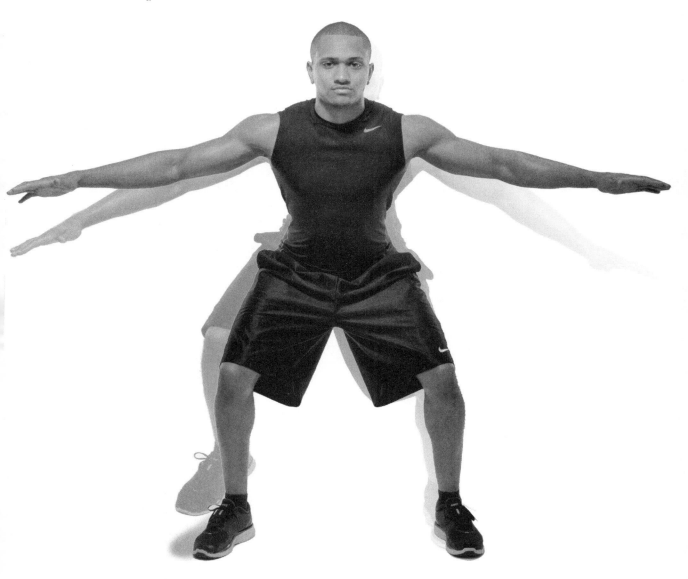

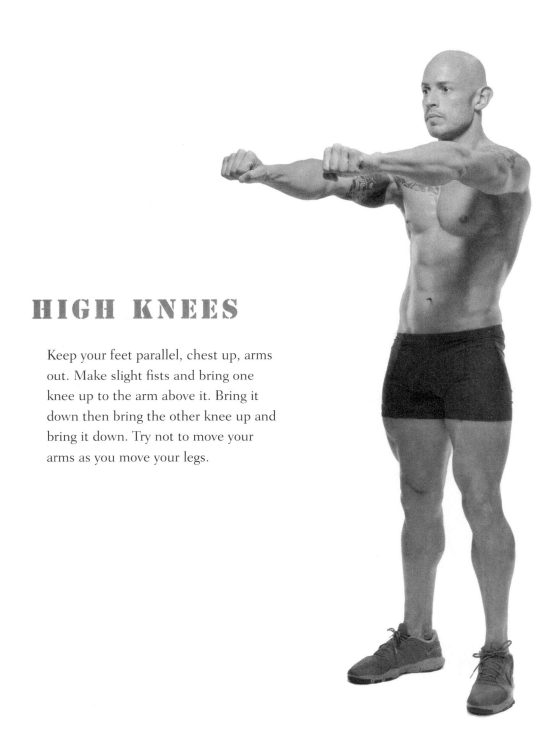

HIGH KNEES

Keep your feet parallel, chest up, arms out. Make slight fists and bring one knee up to the arm above it. Bring it down then bring the other knee up and bring it down. Try not to move your arms as you move your legs.

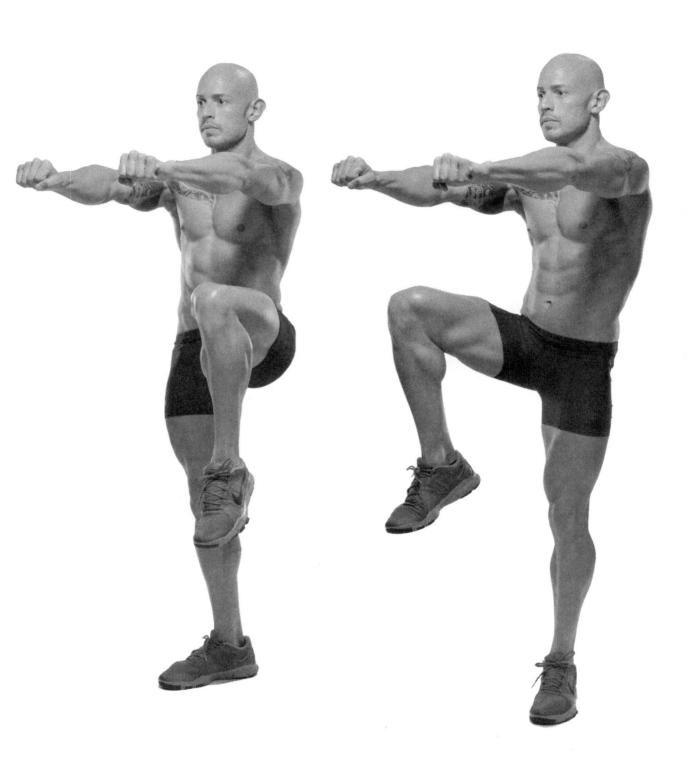

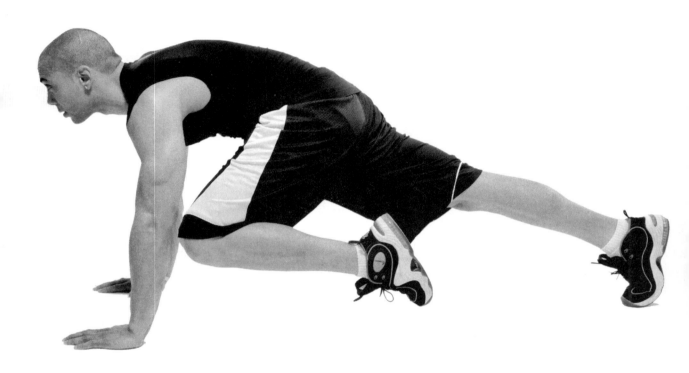

MOUNTAIN CLIMBERS

Start in a push-up position. Keep your hands flat on the floor outside of your legs. Bring one leg forward, then shuffle the legs, alternating from left to right, right to left, at a controlled pace.

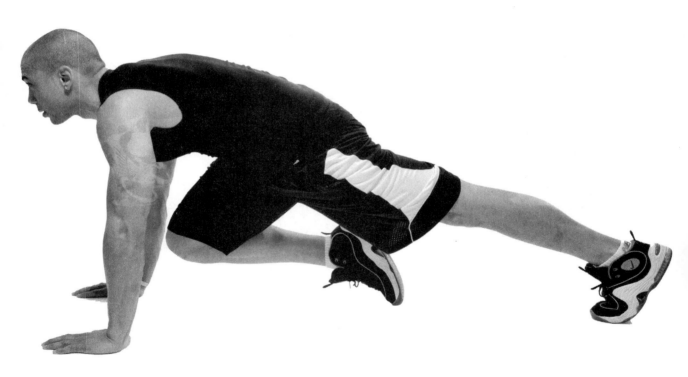

JUMPING JACKS

Start with feet together and arms down by your side.
Jump to open legs and clap hands above head, then
bring arms back down to sides and legs back together.

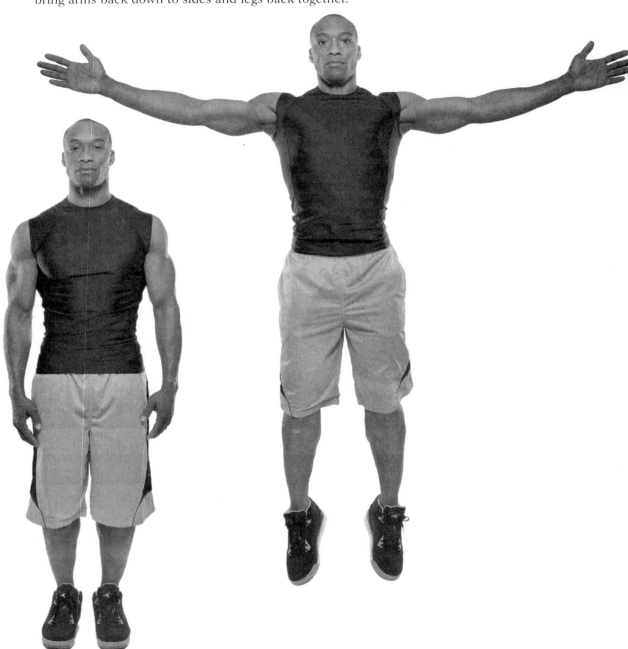

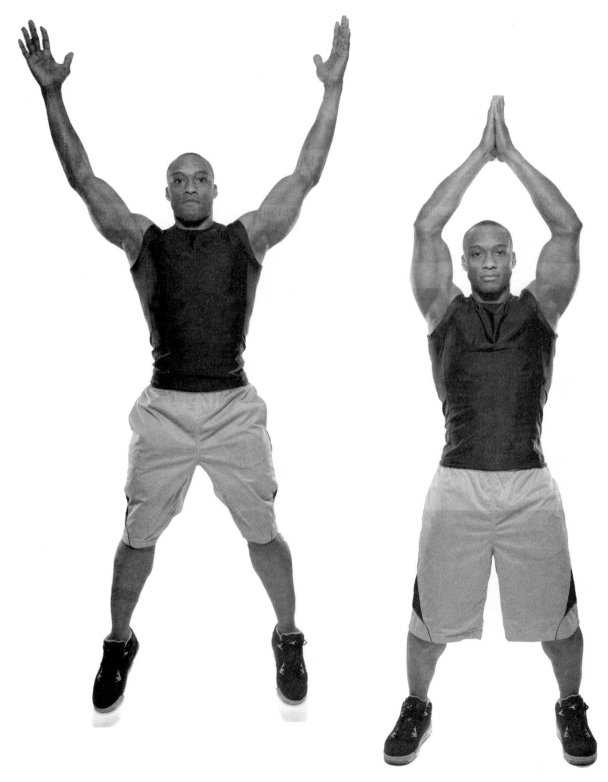

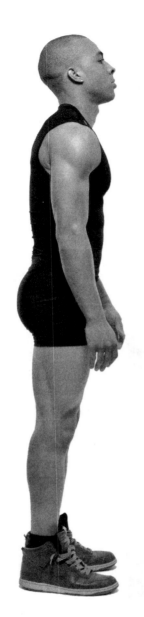
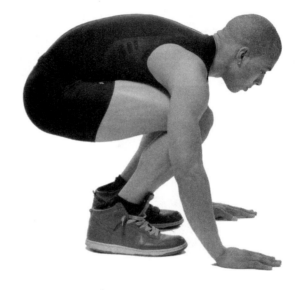

SINGLE-LEG SQUAT THRUSTS

Start in standing position with your feet parallel and arms by your side. Squat down and place hands on the floor, then push one leg back, followed by the other. Now you're in push-up position. Immediately bring the first leg back in, the second leg back in, bend your knees and stand straight up to starting position.

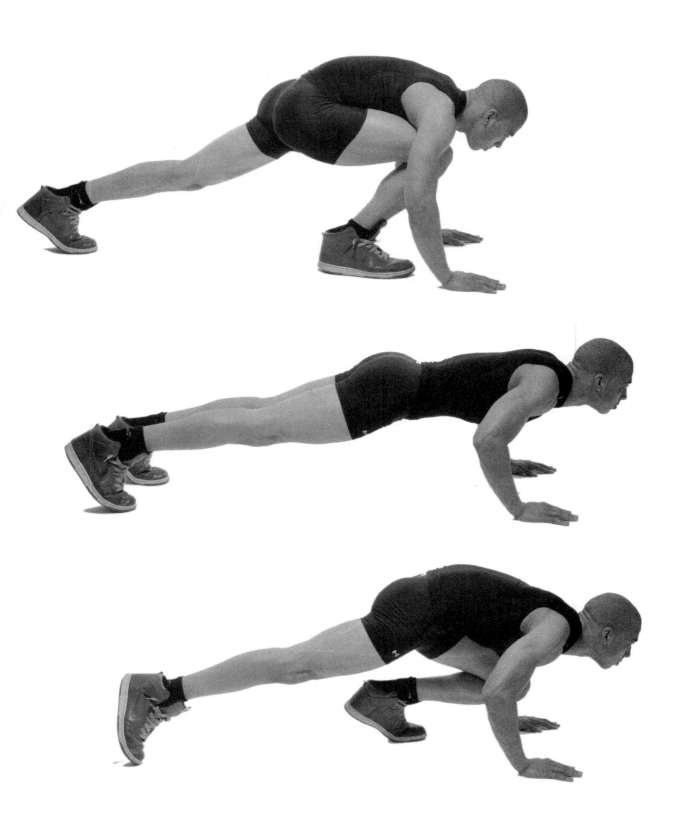

SQUAT THRUSTS

Starting position: Feet parallel. Chest up, arms by your side. Squat down, touch the floor, kick out both legs to straight legs. Now you are in a push-up position. Immediately bend legs back into squat position and stand up straight.

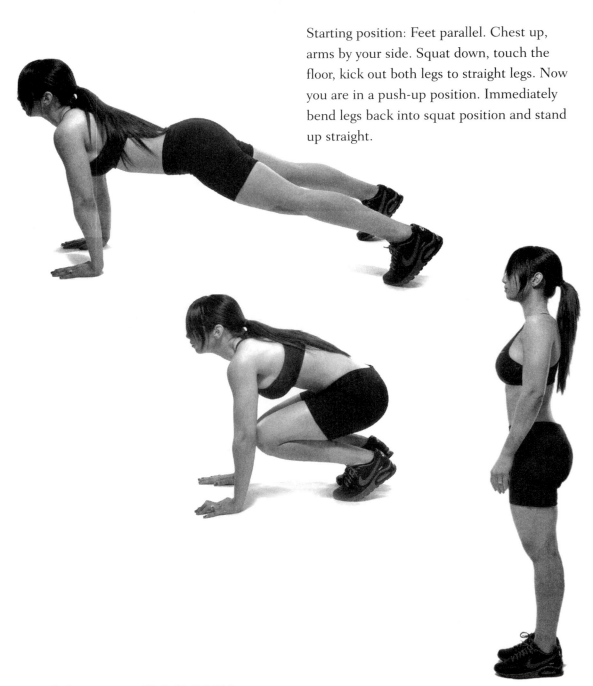

TOE TOUCHES

Start with your legs parallel, hands on your hips and your chest up. Reach down and touch your toes, dropping your head. Return to starting position.

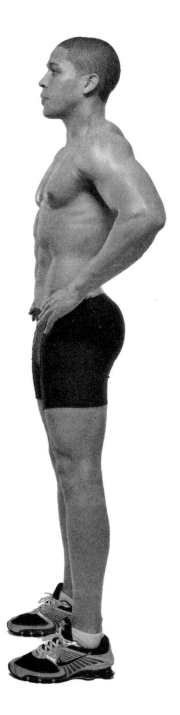

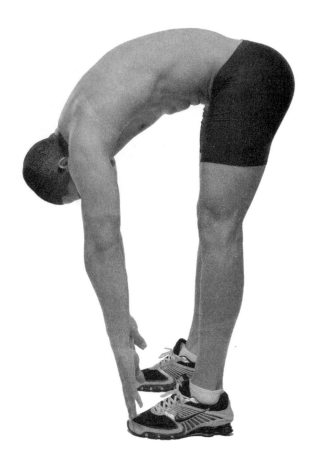

WINDMILL

Start with your legs open wide, arms out to the side and your arms straight. Use your left hand to touch your right toes as your right arm reaches up and back. Return to starting position and reverse it (right hand touches your left toes as your left arm reaches up and back).

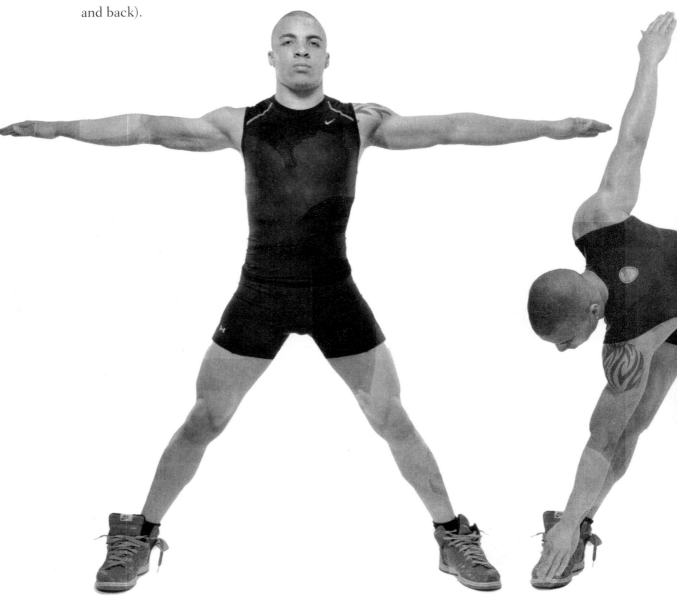

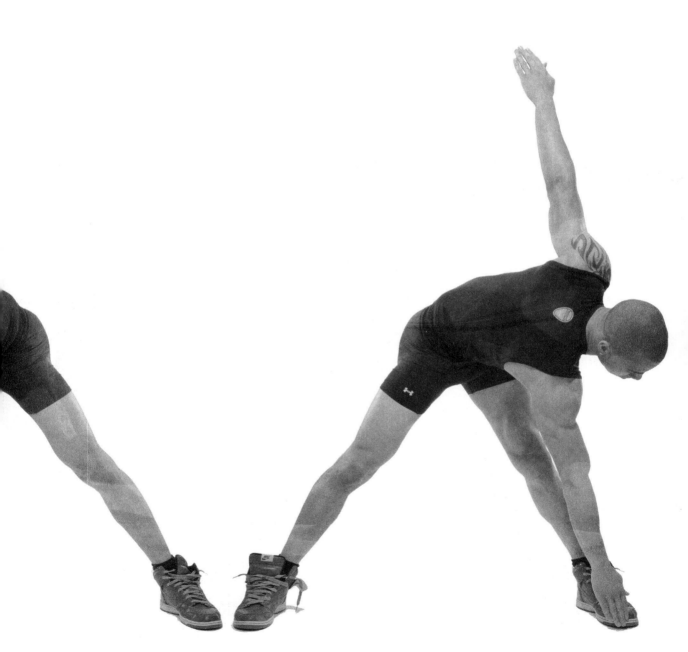

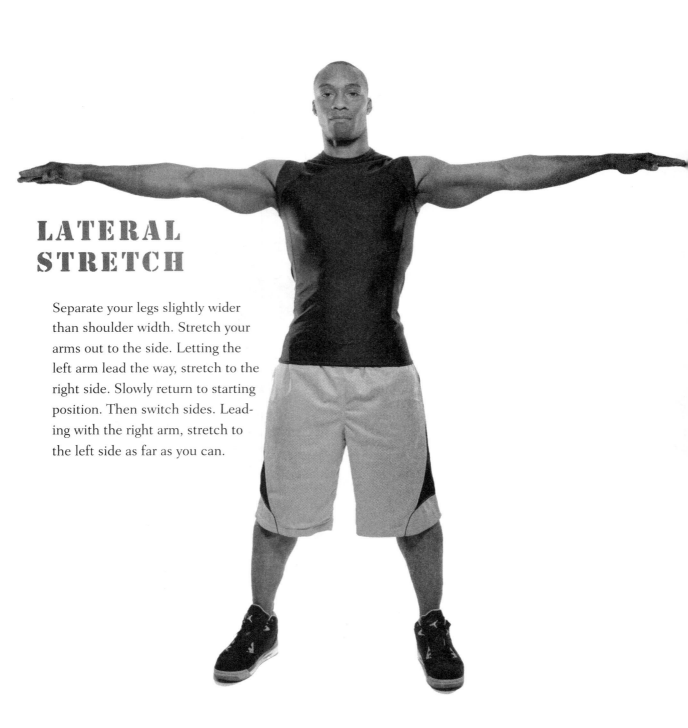

LATERAL STRETCH

Separate your legs slightly wider than shoulder width. Stretch your arms out to the side. Letting the left arm lead the way, stretch to the right side. Slowly return to starting position. Then switch sides. Leading with the right arm, stretch to the left side as far as you can.

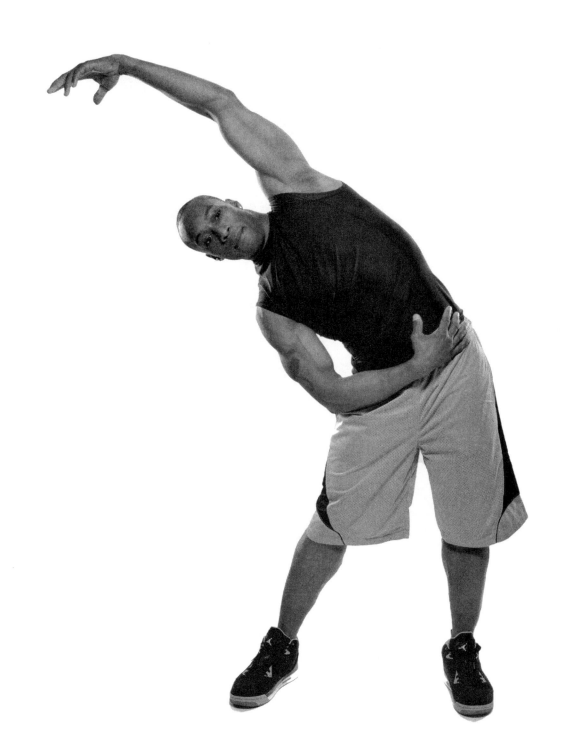

QUAD STRETCH

Stand on both feet. Bring your right leg behind you and use the same arm to pull your heel in toward your hamstrings. Now switch legs. Hold on to a wall if you're unable to balance.

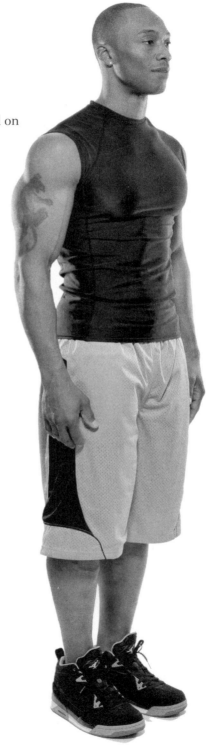

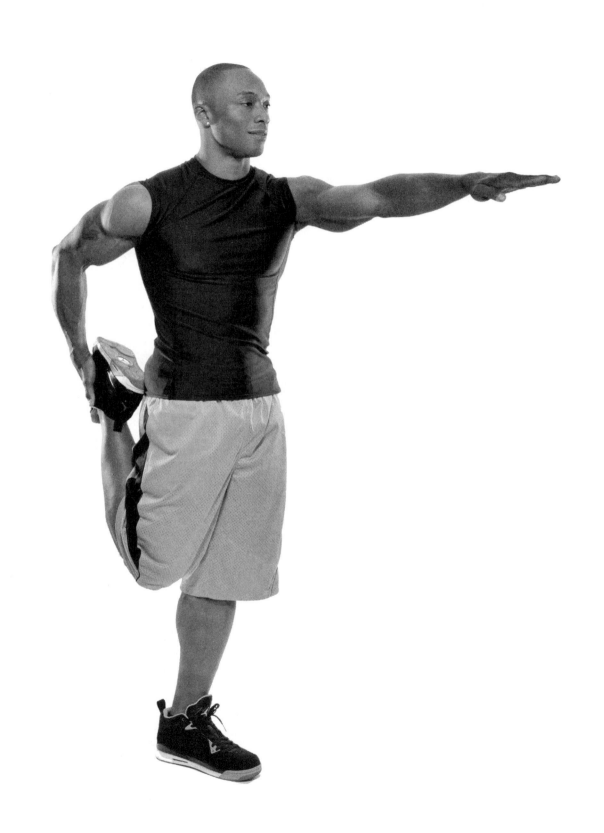

LOWER BACK STRETCH

Lie on your back with your legs bent. Use both arms to pull your
right knee into your chest, keeping your lower back on the floor.
Hold it for a few seconds, then repeat with the opposite leg.

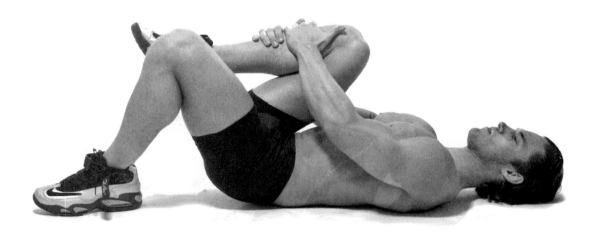

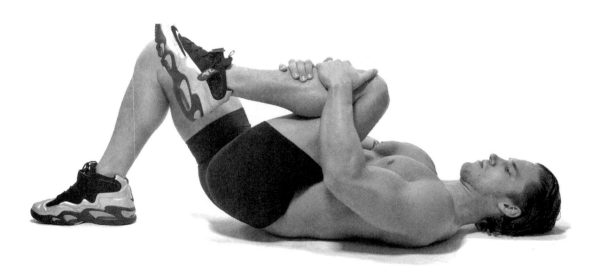

SEATED HAMSTRING STRETCH

Sit down on the floor with your chest up. Lean forward and reach for your toes. Hold that position for a few seconds, keeping your legs as straight as possible. Return to starting position.

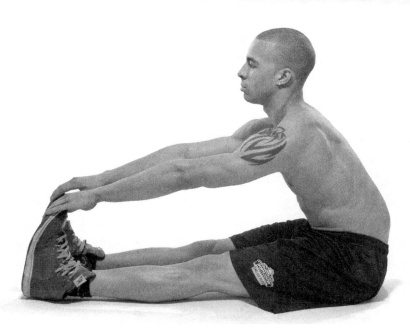

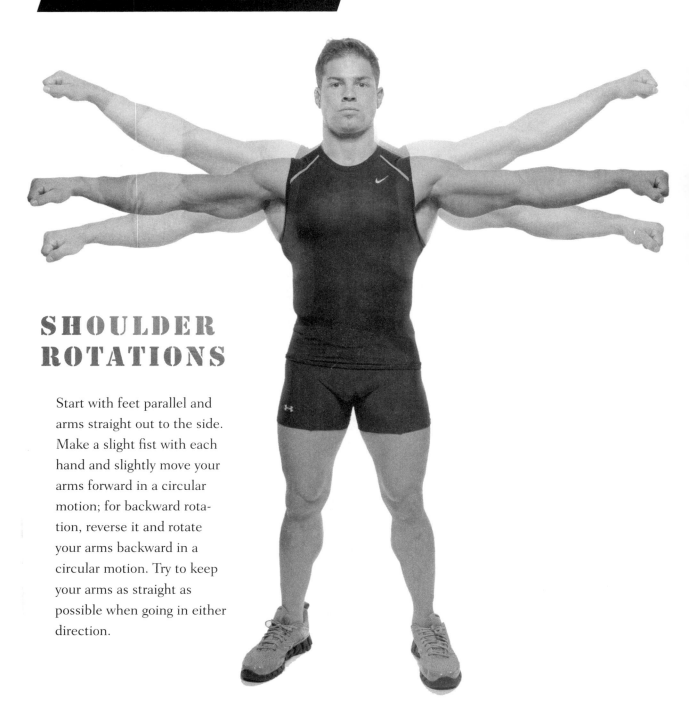

SHOULDER ROTATIONS

Start with feet parallel and arms straight out to the side. Make a slight fist with each hand and slightly move your arms forward in a circular motion; for backward rotation, reverse it and rotate your arms backward in a circular motion. Try to keep your arms as straight as possible when going in either direction.

DIPS

Start by sitting on the floor with your knees bent. You should be on the heels of your feet so that your toes are pointing upward. Place your arms behind you, slightly bent, with your fingers pointing toward your hips. Straighten your arms to bring your bottom off the floor. Bend the elbows slightly and press back up to straight arms. Note: Keep your butt off the floor throughout the exercise.

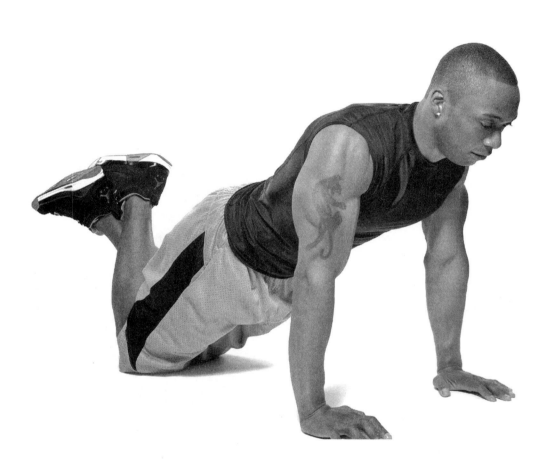

MODIFIED PUSH-UPS

Start in push-up position, but this time with your knees on the ground. Your arms should be slightly wider than your shoulders. Bend the arms to about a 90-degree angle, keeping the weight over your chest as you push back up to straight arms.

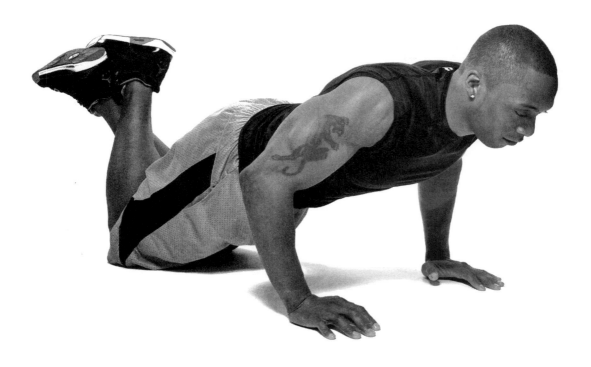

PUSH-UPS

Get into push-up position, with your arms out slightly wider than your shoulders. Keep your body and your core as tight as possible. Bend your elbows and come down to about a 90-degree angle. Push back up to straight arms. It's important to keep your body straight and your core tight during this exercise.

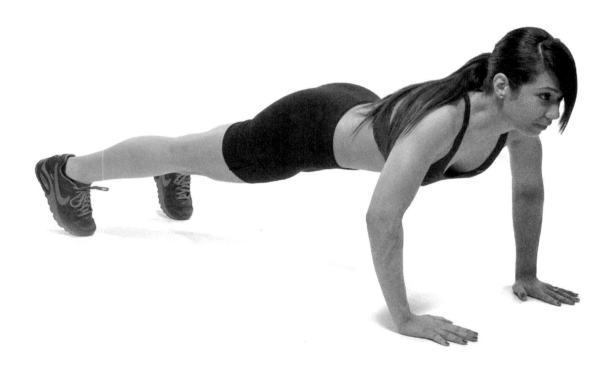

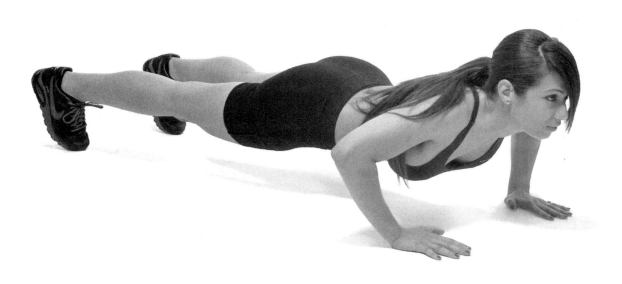

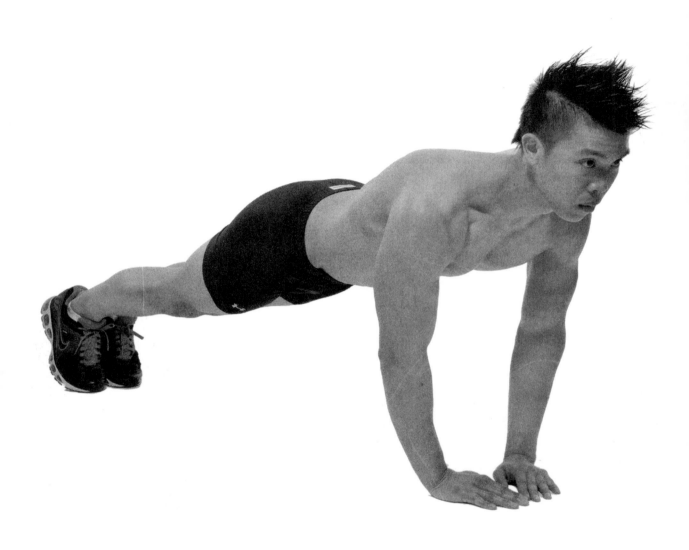

DIAMOND PUSH-UPS

Get into push-up position, bringing your index fingers and thumbs together to form a diamond. Keep the hands very close together. Bend your elbows, bringing your body down as far as you possibly can. Press back up to straighten your arms, keeping your body flat.

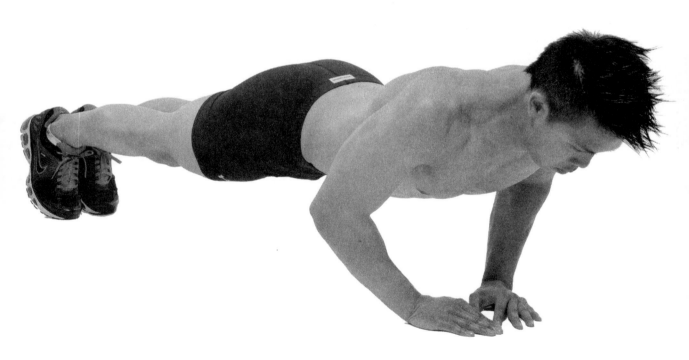

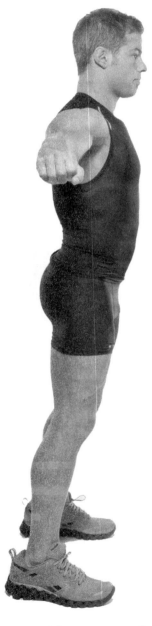

GOOD MORNINGS

Start with your legs slightly wider than your hips, arms open to the side, hands making slight fists. Initiate with your hips, pushing them back as you bring your chest forward. Go forward as far as you can (try to go down to a 90-degree angle) and then slowly squeeze the hips and glutes in as you rise to starting position.

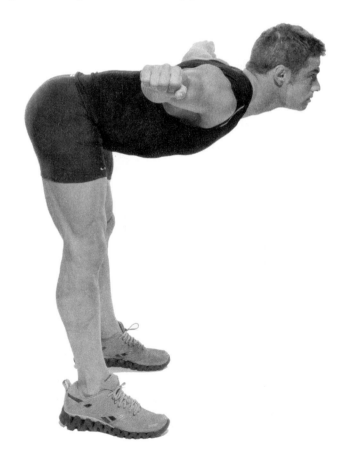

CALF RAISES

Start with your feet flat on the floor, chest up and hands on hips. Press upward with the balls of your feet so that your heels are off the ground, and hold for a few seconds. Slowly return your heels to the floor.

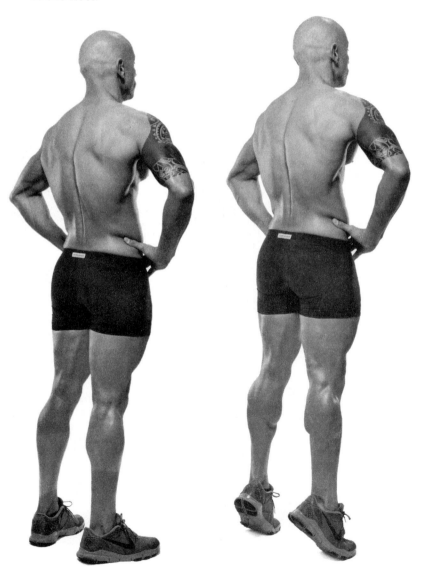

SINGLE-LEG CALF RAISES

Start with your feet parallel and hands on your hips. Bring your left foot behind you and rest it on the back of your right ankle. Push up on the ball of your right foot as far as you can so that your right heel is off the ground, and hold. Bring your right heel down to starting position. Switch legs and repeat. Note: Hold on to a wall if necessary.

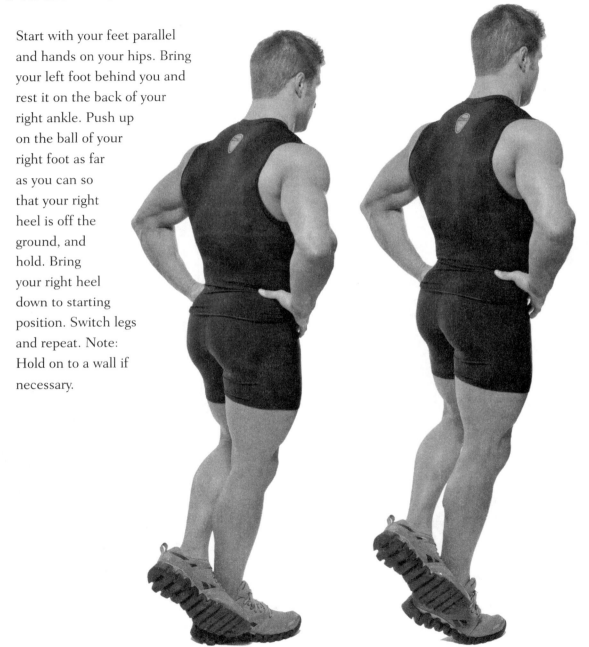

SQUATS

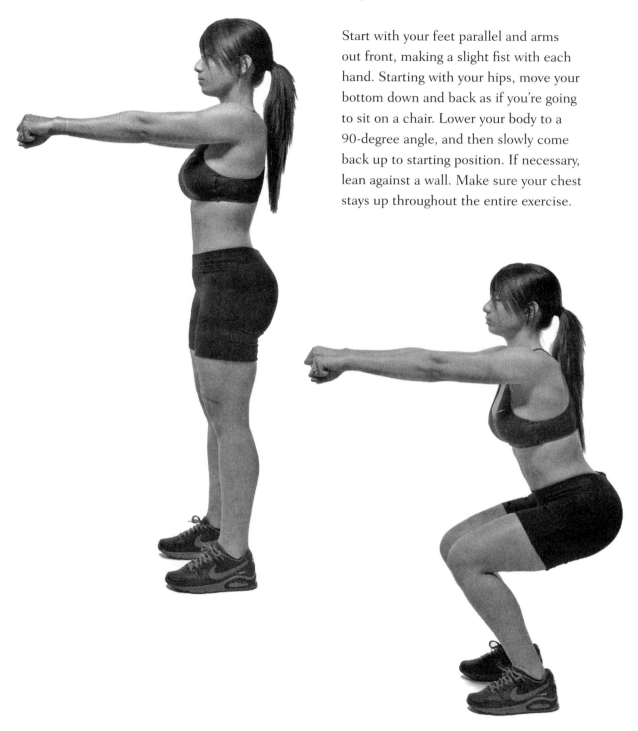

Start with your feet parallel and arms out front, making a slight fist with each hand. Starting with your hips, move your bottom down and back as if you're going to sit on a chair. Lower your body to a 90-degree angle, and then slowly come back up to starting position. If necessary, lean against a wall. Make sure your chest stays up throughout the entire exercise.

LUNGES

Start with your feet parallel, chest up, and hands on hips. Step out on your left leg, keeping your chest up. Bend your knees, slowly lowering your body. Do not let your right knee touch the floor but come as close to it as possible. Slowly rise back up. Repeat, but this time, lead with your right leg.

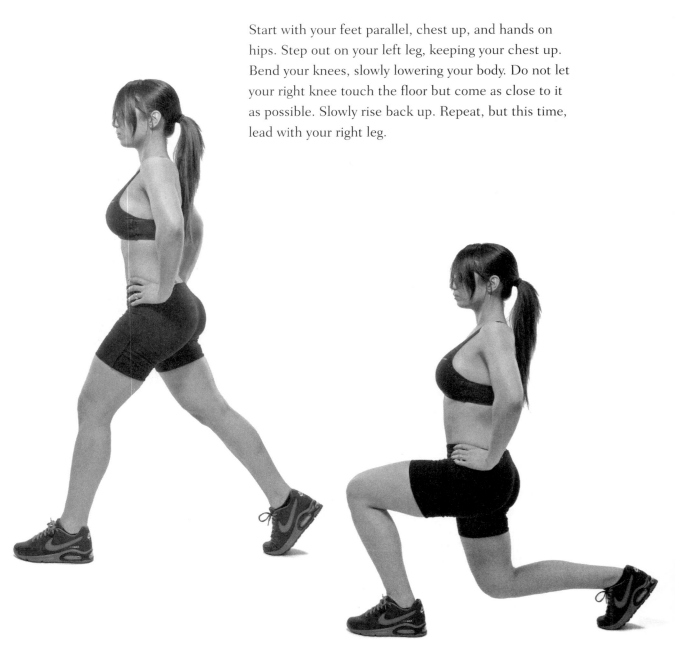

JUMP SQUATS

Start with your knees bent and fingers touching the floor. Jump as high as you can, fingers stretching upward. Return to starting position.

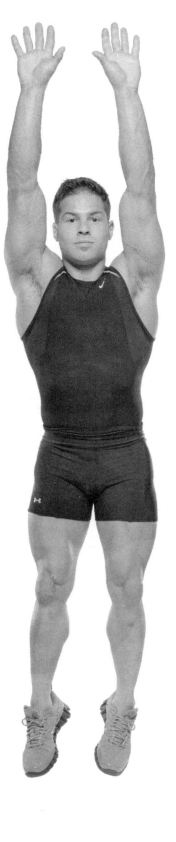

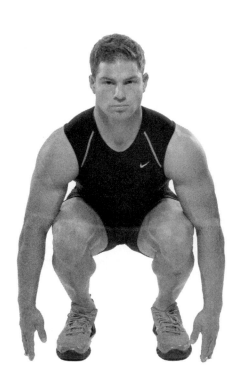

SINGLE-LEG SQUATS

Start with your feet parallel and chest up, with your arms straight out and your hands in slight fists. Bring one leg out straight in front of you, slowly lowering your body on the standing leg and keeping the other leg as straight as possible. Go down as far as you can, hold the position and then slowly return to starting position. Repeat on the opposite leg.

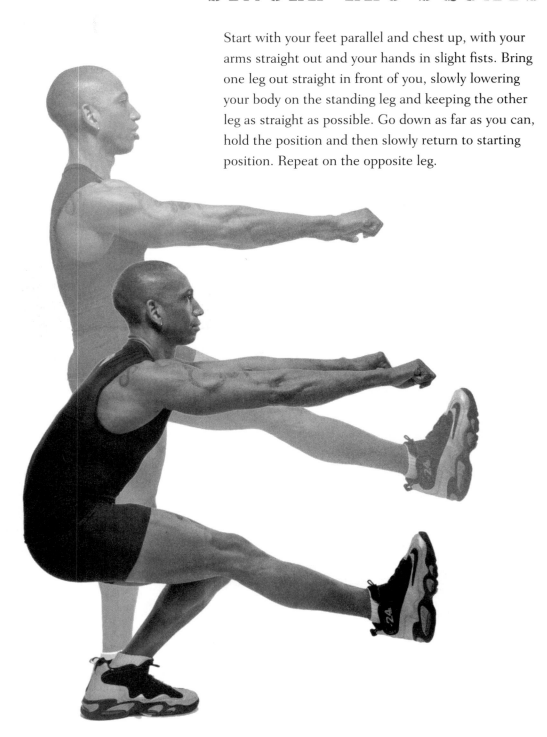

PLANK

Start in a push-up position but with your weight resting on your forearms and your hands in loose fists. Your arms should be as wide as your shoulders. Keep your body straight and your core very tight and hold.

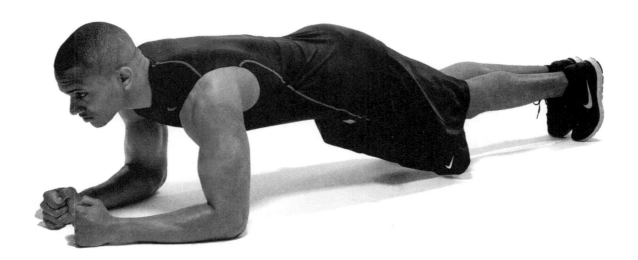

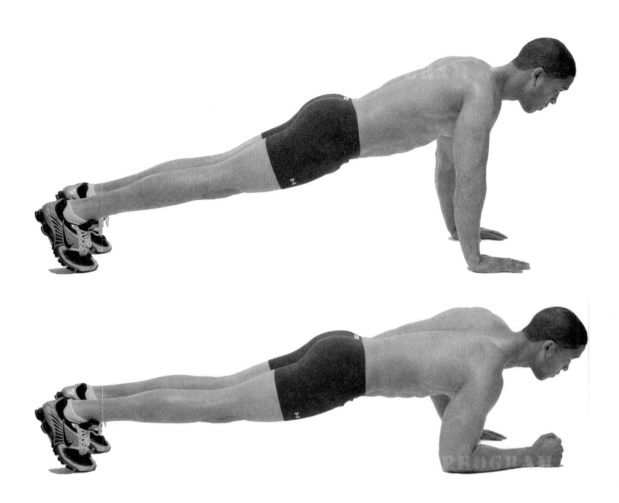

PUSH-UP, PLANK, PUSH-UP

Start in the push-up position. Come down with your right arm and then your left arm so that you're in standard plank position with your weight resting on your forearms. Push up with your right arm and then your left to return to push-up position. Repeat, leading with your left arm.

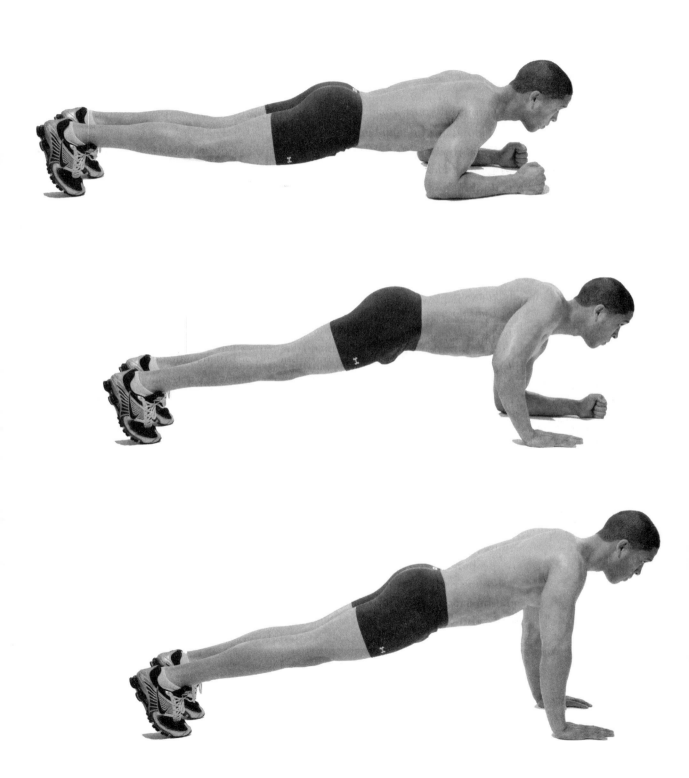

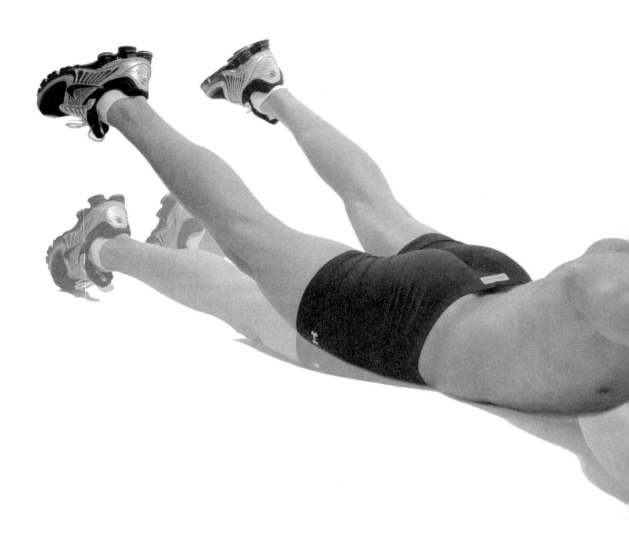

SUPERMAN

Lie on your stomach with your arms reaching out in front and your legs stretched out behind you. Lift your arms and legs off the floor simultaneously, arching your back as much as possible. Hold for ten slow counts and then return to starting position.

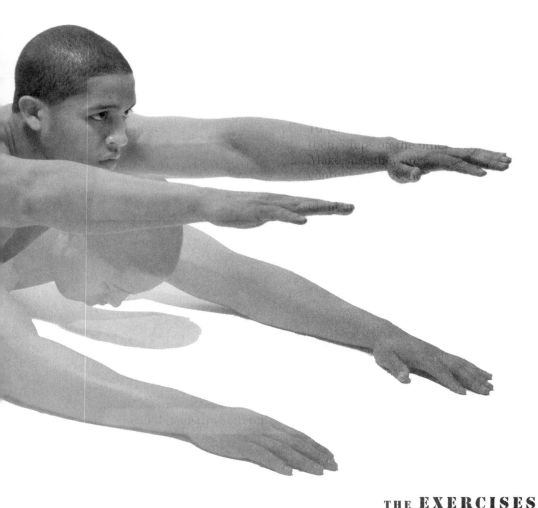

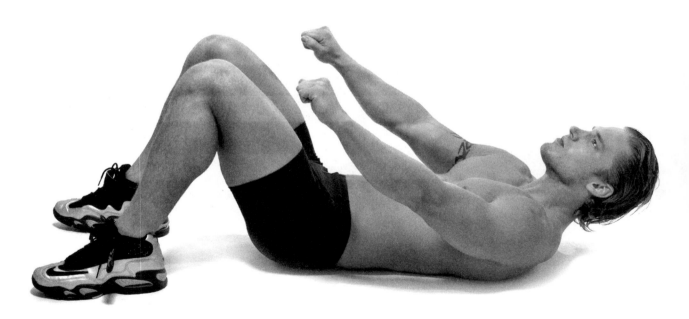

CRUNCHES

Start by lying down on your back, with your legs bent and feet flat on the floor. Raise your arms straight out in front of you and make loose fists with your hands. Come up slightly so that your shoulders and head are off the floor, and then lower your body back to starting position, keeping your shoulders and head off the floor throughout the set. Note: The crunch should initiate with your core, not your neck. Straining your neck can lead to injury.

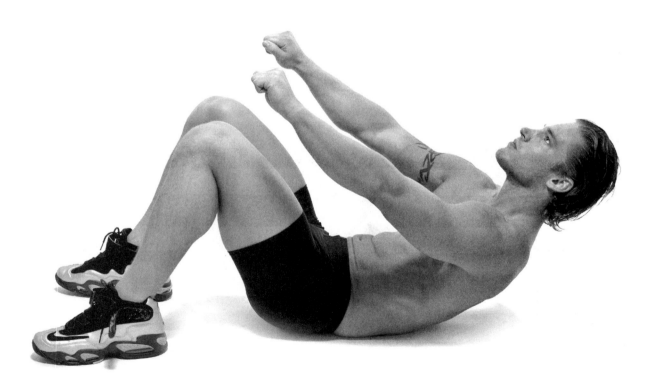

TABLETOP CRUNCHES

Start in standard crunch position, raising your feet off the ground so that your legs form a 90-degree angle (a tabletop). Raise your arms straight out in front of you and make loose fists with your hands. Come up slightly so that your shoulders and head are off the floor, and then lower your body back to starting position. Keep your head and shoulders off the floor throughout the set.

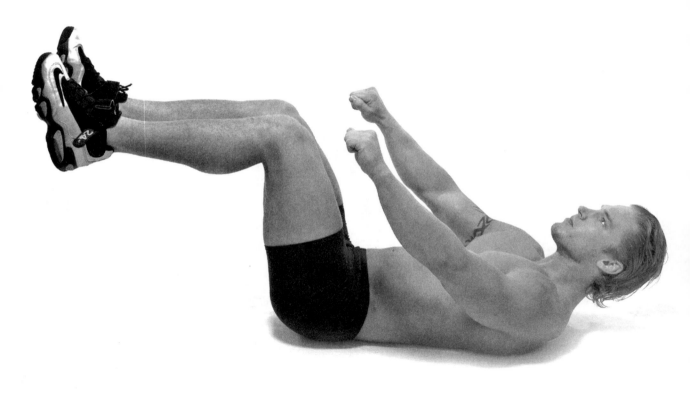

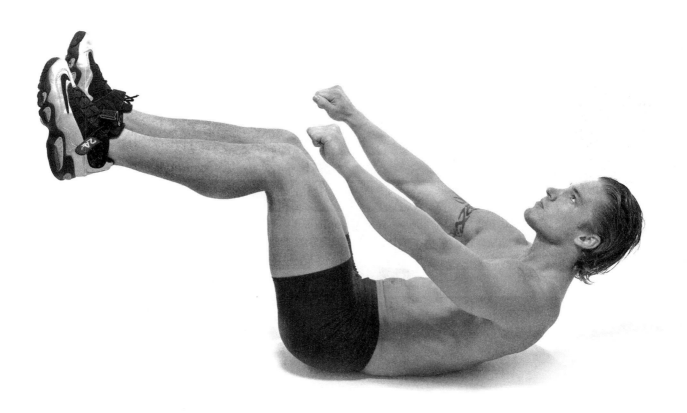

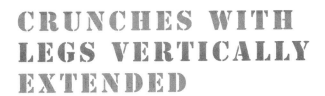

CRUNCHES WITH LEGS VERTICALLY EXTENDED

Start by lying down on your back, with your legs straight up in the air. Come up slightly, keeping your arms outside your legs and your legs extended straight up. Lower your body back down. Remember that the crunch should initiate with your core, not your neck.

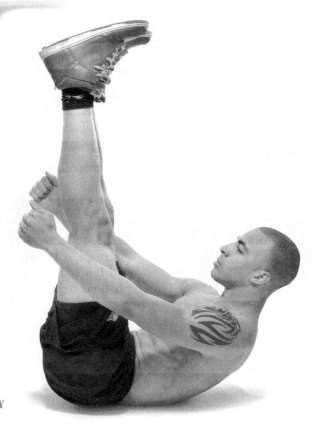

FLUTTER KICKS

Lie on your back with your arms down by your side. Bring your feet slightly off the floor, keeping the legs as straight as possible, and flutter the legs up and down. Be sure to keep your lower back as relaxed as possible. Note: Your feet should stay off the floor throughout the set.

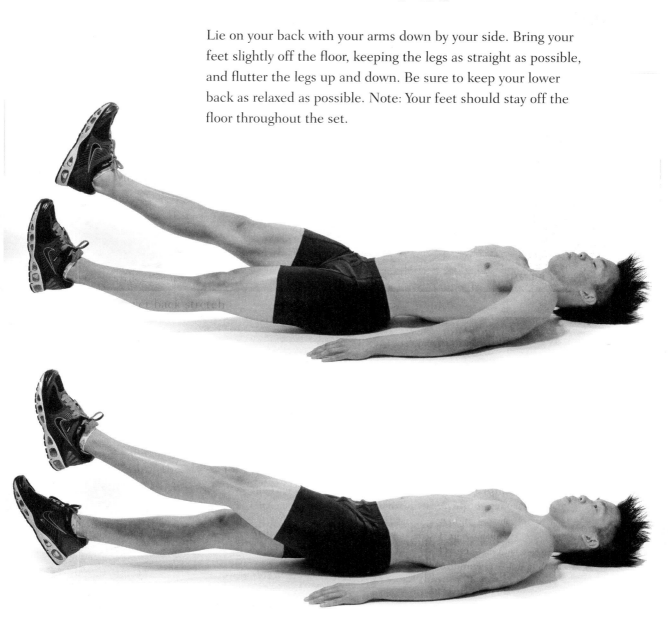

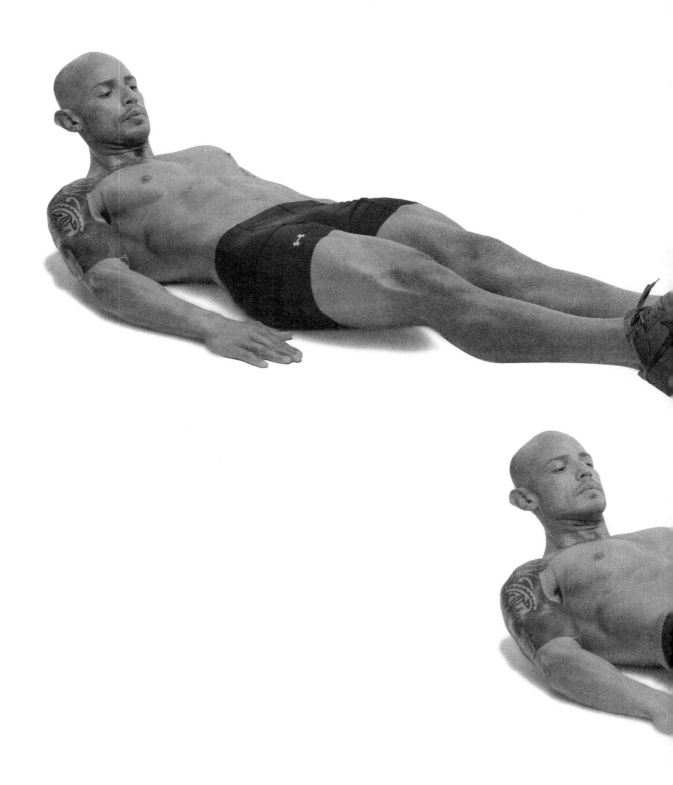

SCISSORS

Lie on your back and bring your feet up slightly off the floor. Slightly open and close your legs, touching your heels together as fast as possible. Note: Your feet should stay off the floor throughout the set.

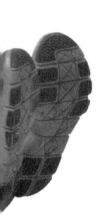
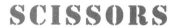
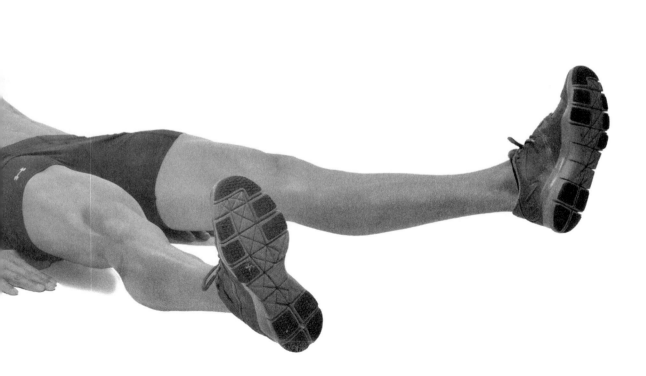

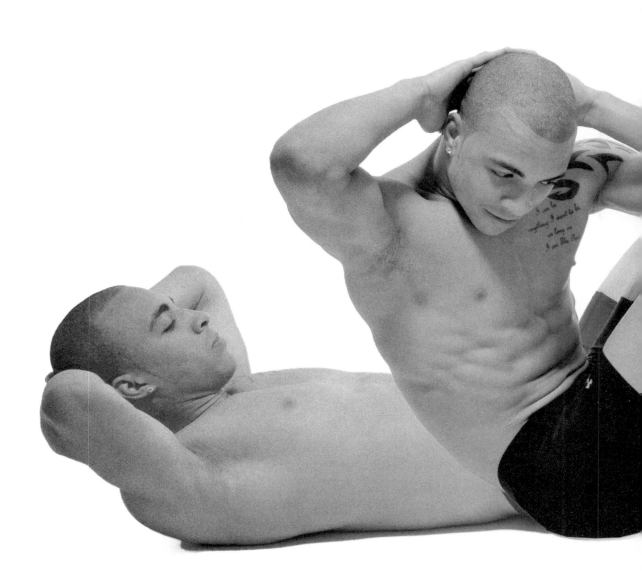

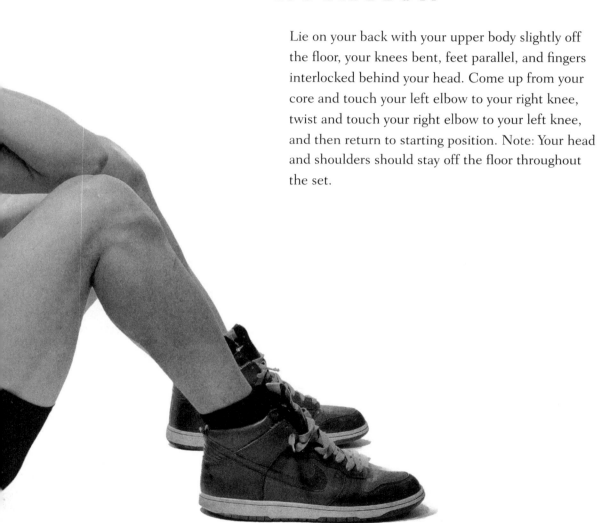

SIT-UPS WITH ROTATION

Lie on your back with your upper body slightly off the floor, your knees bent, feet parallel, and fingers interlocked behind your head. Come up from your core and touch your left elbow to your right knee, twist and touch your right elbow to your left knee, and then return to starting position. Note: Your head and shoulders should stay off the floor throughout the set.

ASSISTED SIT-UPS WITH ROTATION

Lie on your back with your upper body slightly off the floor, your knees bent, feet parallel and fingers interlocked behind your head. Have a partner hold your feet down. Come up from your core and touch your left elbow to your right knee, twist and touch your right elbow to your left knee, and then return to starting position.

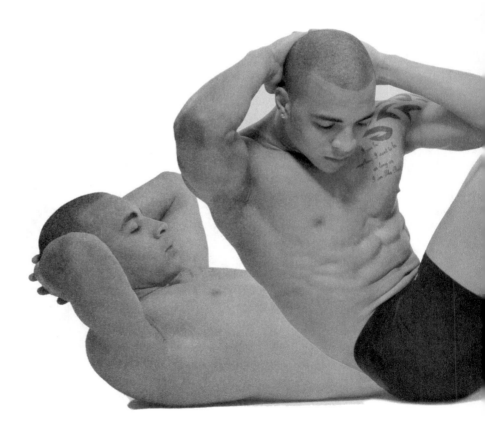

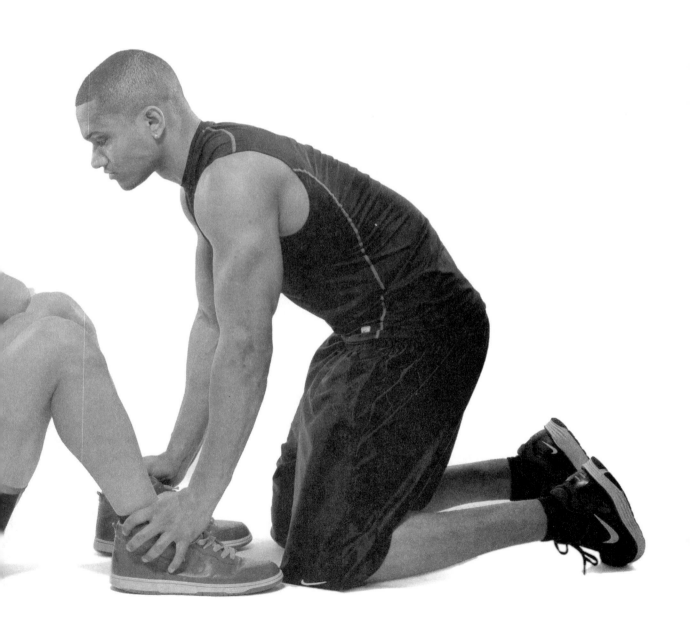

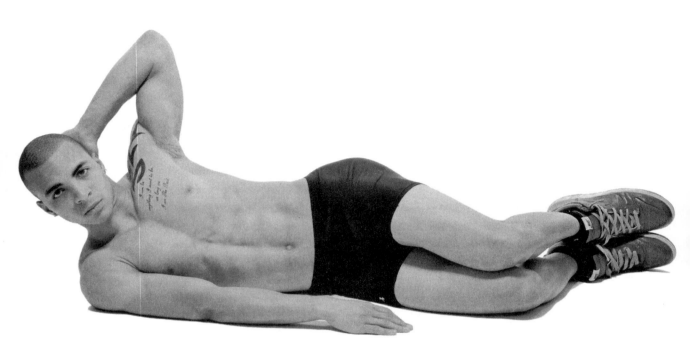

SIDE CRUNCHES

Lie on your right side with your legs bent, left arm
behind your head and your right hand by your right side
or on the floor. Squeeze your abdominals to come up off
the floor and slowly return to starting position. Repeat on
left side.

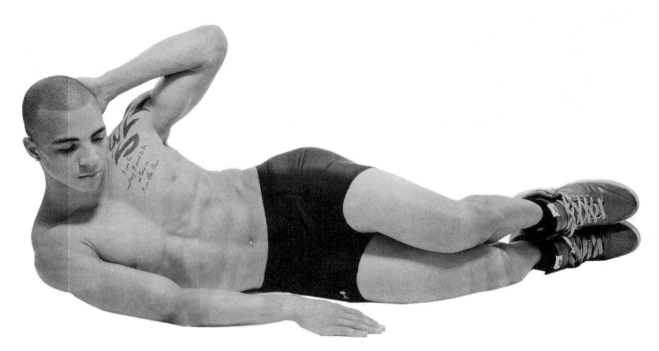

THE AIRPLANE

Lie on your back and bring your legs off the floor so that
your knees are bent in a tabletop position (90-degree angle).
Cross your arms over your torso. Raise your torso off the floor,
simultaneously opening up your arms to the sides, like wings.
Balance on your tailbone for a few seconds, then return to
starting position by lowering your torso back down and cross-
ing your arms across your chest. Your feet should remain off
the floor in a tabletop position.

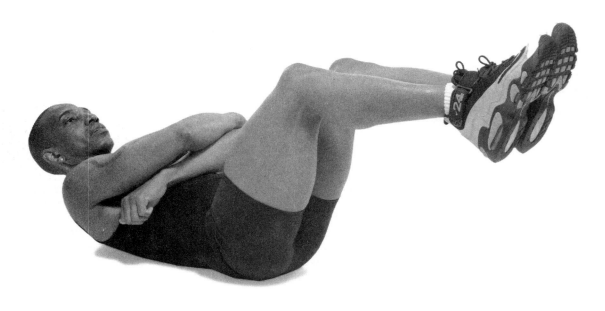

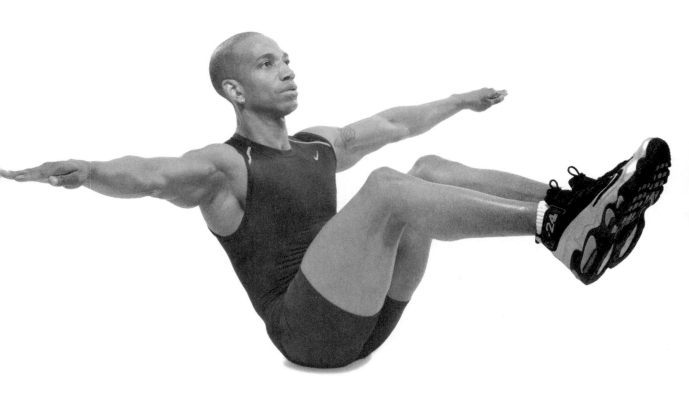

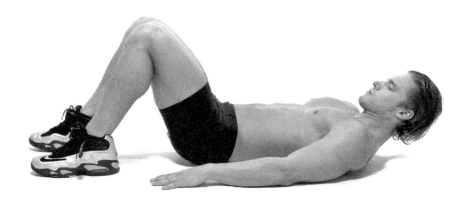

TUCK IN, PUSH UP, TUCK IN, PUSH OUT

Lie flat on your back with your knees bent and your arms facedown on the floor. Bend your legs in to push your bottom up off the floor, straightening your legs slightly as you push your legs and bottom straight up in the air. Bend your legs back in and press out to straighten your legs. Repeat.

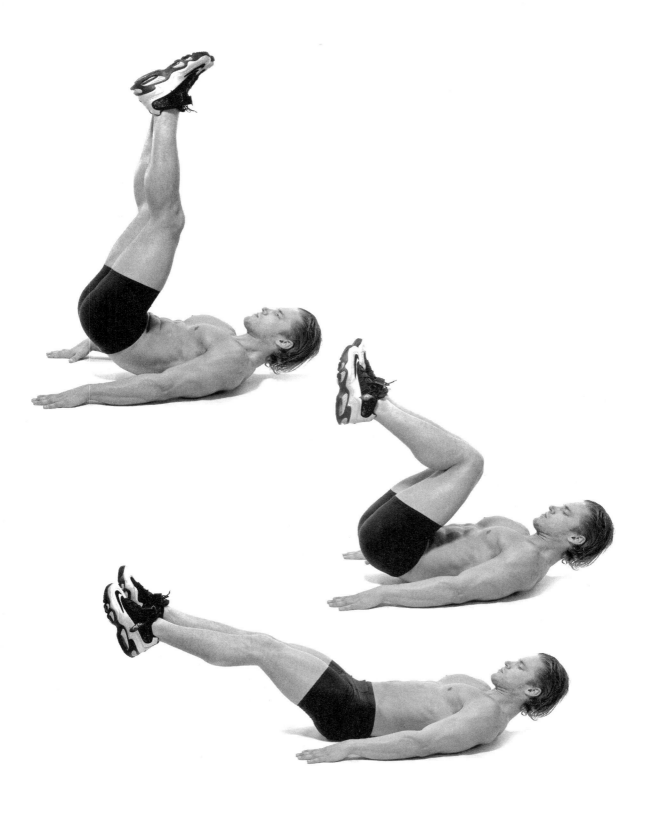

THE LASALLE

Lie on your back with your legs bent, feet on the floor, and knees together. Extend your right leg straight with both knees touching. Raise up with your upper body as far as possible (ideally sitting up on your tailbone), reaching forward with your arms. Extend your left leg so that both legs are now straight. Hold this position for a few seconds. Bend your left leg in, and hold for a few seconds. Return to start position and switch to opposite side, extending your left leg to start.

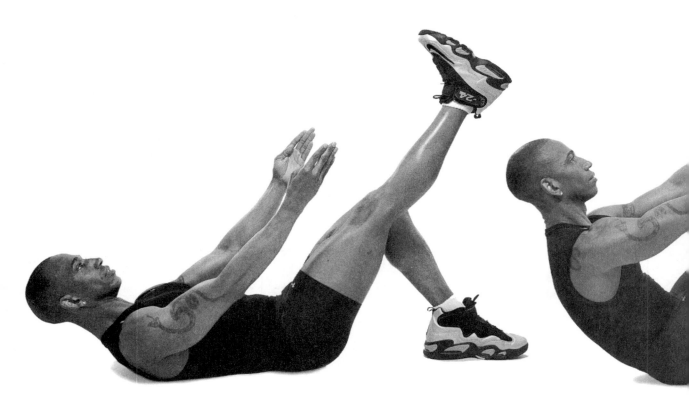

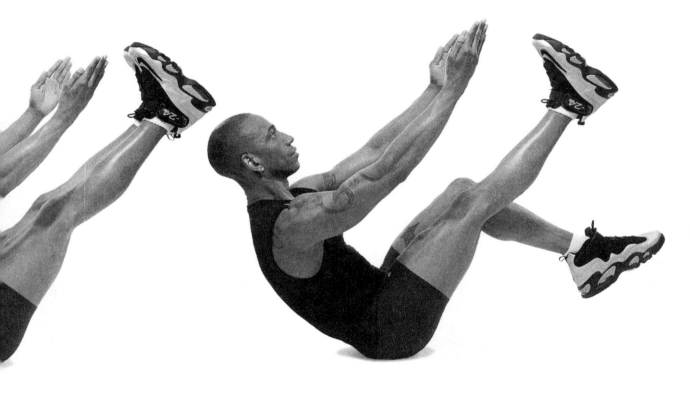

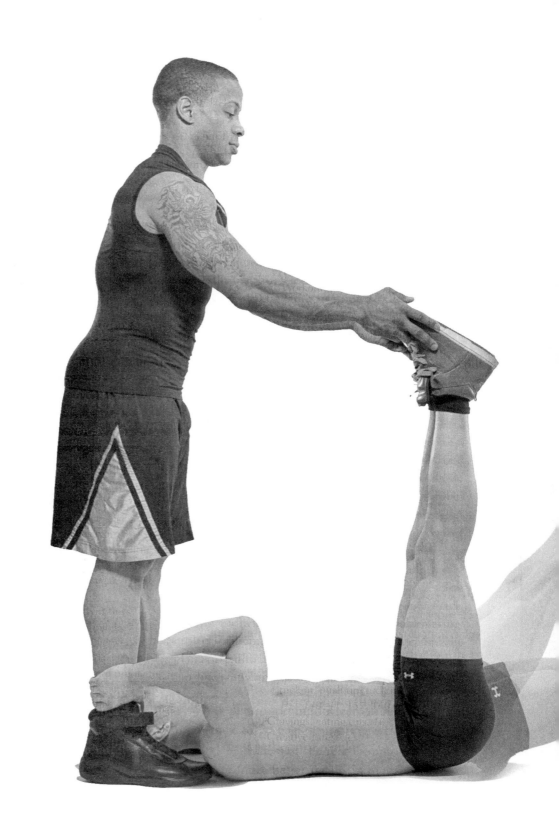

LEG THROW-DOWNS

Lie on the floor with your legs straight out, arms behind your head, holding on to your partner's ankles. Keeping your legs as straight as possible, bring them straight up to your partner. As your partner pushes your legs down, try to control your legs as much as possible. Then return to starting position. You should let your legs go down as close to the floor as possible without touching it.

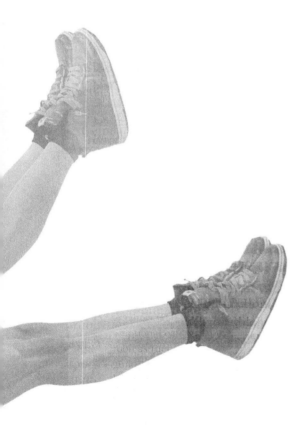

BICYCLES

Lie on your back with your feet off the floor in a tabletop position. Keep your fingers interlocked behind your neck and your elbows open. Come up and twist, touching your right elbow to your left knee and then your left elbow to your right knee. Note: Keep your head and shoulders off the floor throughout the set.

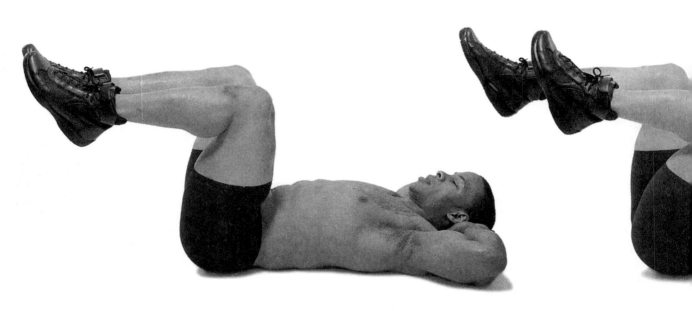

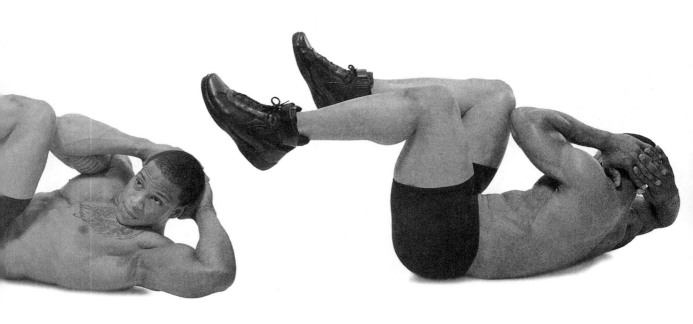

CURL IN, RELEASE OUT

Lie on your back with your knees bent and your feet on the floor.
With your fingers interlocked behind your neck, curl in
(bringing your knees to your elbows) and release out
(straightening your legs).

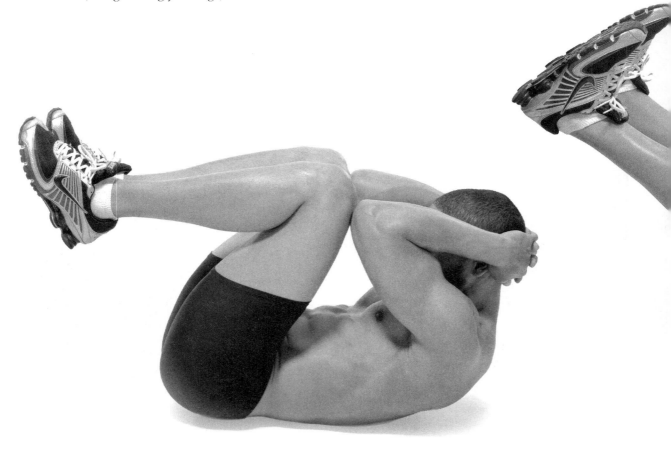

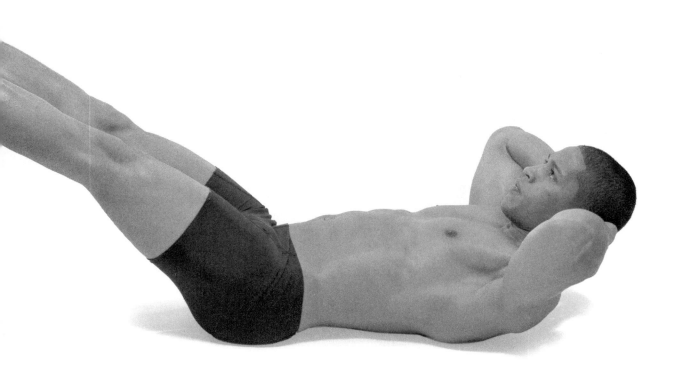

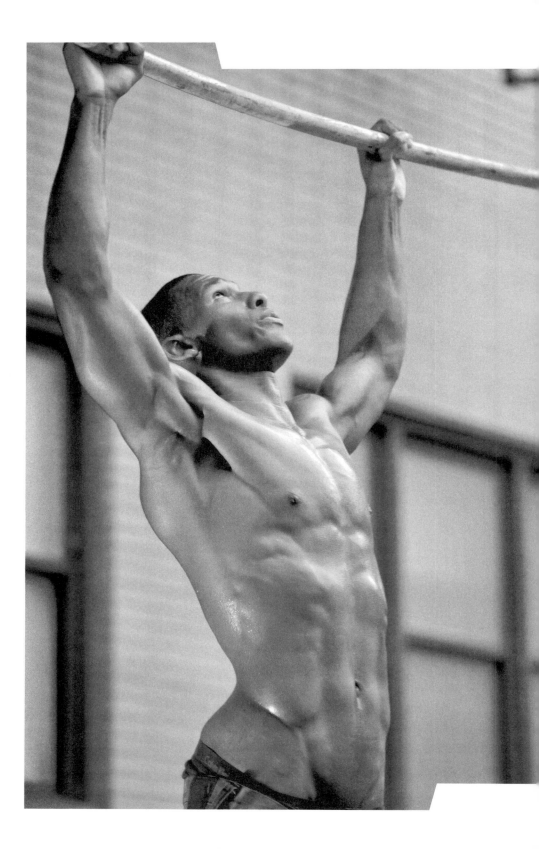

THE
WORKOUT

A 90-DAY PROGRAM
WITH THREE PHASES

BEGINNER PROGRAM

The Beginner Program is for those who have never trained before or who haven't trained consistently within the last six months. In this program, you will complete Phase 1, Phase 2, and Phase 3 for thirty days each. Each phase is designed to be completed straight through, from start to finish, and can be performed from one to five days a week, depending on your fitness level.

Day 1–30: Complete Phase 1

Day 31–60: Complete Phase 2

Day 61–90: Complete Phase 3

INTERMEDIATE PROGRAM

The Intermediate Program is for those who have been consistently participating in some sort of physical training for a year. Intermediates will begin by completing Phase 2 from one to five days a week for forty-five days, and then finish up by completing Phase 3 for one to five days a week for the final forty-five days.

Day 1–45: Complete Phase 2

Day 46–90 Complete Phase 3

ADVANCED PROGRAM

The Advanced Program is for those who have been strength training consistently for the last two years and are looking for a new challenge. Advanced trainers will complete Phase 3 from one to five days a week for the full ninety-day period.

Day 1–90: Complete Phase 3

Note: Asterisks (*) in the workout plan indicate Super Sets. A Super Set is a combination of two or more exercises where, instead of completing all of the sets for the first exercise and then moving on to the second exercise, you move immediately to the next exercise after completing the first set without taking a break until all the sets for all the exercises are completed.

PHASE 1

Warm-up

EXERCISE	REPS	SETS
Running	10 minutes	1
High knees	8 (on each leg)	4
Jumping jacks	5	4
Quick feet	60 seconds	1

Stretches

STRETCH	REPS	SETS
Toe touches	12	1
Lateral stretch	2 times on each side	1
Windmill	10 (on each side)	1
Quad stretch	2 times on each leg	1

Workout

EXERCISE	REPS	SETS
Calf raises	10	3
Single-leg squat thrusts	10	1
Shoulder rotation	10	3 sets forward and 3 sets backward
Plank	Hold for slow 10 count.	3

EXERCISE	REPS	SETS
Push-ups or modified push-ups	10	3
Dips	5	3
Superman	Hold for slow 10 count.	3
Crunches	10	3
Tabletop crunches	10	3
Side crunches	10	3
Flutter kicks	10	3
Scissors	10	3
Bicycles	10 (on each side)	3
Squats	10 (Hold for a slow 10 count in your seated position at the end of each set.)	3
Lunges	10 (Do 5 reps on one leg, then 5 reps on the other leg. Make sure they are 5 continuous reps, not alternating from one leg to the next.)	3
Quick feet	60 seconds	1
Jumping jacks	5	4

Cooldown

STRETCH

Lower back stretch

Seated hamstring stretch

PHASE 2

Warm-up

EXERCISE	REPS	SETS
Running	10 minutes	1
High knees	10 (on each leg)	4
Jumping jacks	10	4
Quick feet	60 seconds	1
Mountain climbers	10	4

Stretches

STRETCH	REPS	SETS
Good mornings	8	1
Toe touches	10	1
Lateral stretch	2 times each side	1
Windmill	10 (on each side)	1
Quad stretch	2 times on each leg	1

Workout

EXERCISE	REPS	SETS
Calf raises*	10	3
Single-leg calf raises*	10 (on each foot)	3
Single-leg squats	2 (on each leg)	3
Single-leg squat thrusts	10	1

EXERCISE	REPS	SETS
Squat thrusts	10	1
Shoulder rotations	10	3 sets forward and 3 sets backward
Plank*	Hold for slow 10 count.	3
Push-up, plank, push-up*	10	3
Push-ups*	10	3
Dips*	10	3
Superman*	Hold for slow 10 count.	3
Sit-ups with rotation	10 (on each side)	2
Leg throw-downs	10	1
Crunches	20	1
Tabletop crunches	20	1
Crunches with legs vertically extended	20	1
Side crunches	30 (on each side)	1
Flutter kicks	40	1
Scissors	40	1
Tuck in, push up, tuck in, push out	10	1
Bicycles	10 slow reps, followed immediately by 20 fast reps	4
Curl in, release out	10	1
Squats*	10 (Hold for a slow 10 count in your seated position at the end of each set.)	3

2 EXERCISE	REPS	SETS
Lunges*	10 reps on one leg, then 10 reps on the other	3
Jump squats*	10 (Hold for a slow 10 count in your seated position at the end of each set.)	3

Cooldown

STRETCH

Lower back stretch

Seated hamstring stretch

PHASE 3

Warm-up

EXERCISE	REPS	SETS
Running	10 minutes	1
High knees	10 (on each leg)	5
Jumping jacks	10	6
Quick feet	90 seconds	1
Mountain climbers	10	6

Stretches

STRETCH	REPS	SETS
Good mornings	10	1
Toe touches	12	1
Lateral stretch	2 times on each side	1
Windmill	12 (on each side)	1
Quad stretch	2 times on each leg	1

Workout

EXERCISE	REPS	SETS
Calf raises*	10	3
Single-leg calf raises*	10 (on each foot)	3
Single-leg squats	5 (on each leg)	3

3

EXERCISE	REPS	SETS
Single-leg squat thrusts	15	1
Squat thrusts	20	1
Plank*	Hold for slow 10 count.	3
Push-up, plank, push-up*	10	3
Push-ups*	10	3
Dips*	10	3
Diamond push-ups*	10	3
Superman	Hold for slow 10 count.	3
Leg throw-downs	20	1
Sit-ups with rotation	10 (on each side)	2
The airplane	10 (Hold for slow 10 count on last rep.)	1
Crunches	20	1
Tabletop crunches	20	1
Crunches with legs vertically extended	20	1
Side crunches	40 (40 reps on each side)	1
Flutter kicks	60	1
Scissors	60	1
Tuck in, push up, tuck in, push out	20	1
The LaSalle	For each set, 1 rep with the right leg extended and 1 rep with the left leg extended	3
Bicycles	10 slow reps followed immediately by 20 fast reps	5
Curl in, release out	15	1

EXERCISE	REPS	SETS
Squats*	10 (Hold for a slow 10 count in your seated position at the end of each set.)	3
Lunges*	10 reps on one leg, then switch to the next leg and do 10 reps	3
Jump squats*	10 (Hold for a slow 10 count in your seated position at the end of each set.)	3
Quick feet	90 seconds	1
Mountain climbers	10	6

Cooldown

STRETCH

Lower back stretch

Seated hamstring stretch

TEN EATING TIPS

FOOD, OF COURSE, is a major factor in changing your body when you're not being physically active . . . but once you start exercising, it becomes less important and begins to have less power over you. That's what's so amazing about exercising: You can offset food, age and genetics. The more you exercise, the less important genetics and food become. So, if you're ready to get that bangin' body and embark on a lifetime of health through regular exercise, here are some eating tips that are realistic and doable for anyone who is ready to commit to being physically active.

1. Eat a balanced diet (protein, carbs, fat). Keep it basic and simple.

2. Get your protein from chicken, fish, meats and eggs instead of protein shakes. These are natural sources of protein, which is always the best.

3. **Eat three meals a day.** Keep it simple. Adding more meals is actually going to make you only fatter.

4. Drink a lot of **water.** It tastes good, it's free, it's good for your skin and it fills you up. Most of all, it has zero calories.

5. Eat your larger meals earlier in the day, so that you can **burn off the calories before bedtime.**

6. **Eat smaller portions.** You do not have to eat until you're stuffed or your plate is empty.

7. **Eat slowly.** You'll eat less and you'll enjoy your food more.

8. Do not deprive yourself of a food that you really want to eat. **This will make you crave it only more.**

9. **Do not feel guilty after eating;** do extra exercises to burn it all off, and no one will ever know.

10. Do not use food as a psychological crutch or a reward. Food is for energy. It's not your lover, your companion or your best friend. It's also not your enemy. **Food is fuel—** it's necessary and you should enjoy it.

FINAL THOUGHTS

AT THE END OF THE DAY, we all want to look and feel good; how we get there is still debatable. But after fifteen years of shaping minds and bodies, we're convinced that placing the focus on physical activities is a more effective way of creating a fit America. As a nation struggling to keep the pounds off, we must open our minds to a new approach, particularly if the old ones are obviously not working. To make fitness a lifestyle, we must set simple, attainable daily goals for ourselves, which must include physical activities. Remember: We can all create our own bangin' body if we commit ourselves to the physical work and effort that is necessary. The more effort you give, the more bangin' you will look and feel. It's all up to you. Your physical destiny is in your hands.

1. The price for our advanced technology in the USA is the fat around our stomach. Despite how great it is, technology has created a lazy society.

2. Food is not the enemy. You can eat whatever you want— in moderation—if you're willing to burn it off with exercise.

3. A good workout does not discriminate against age, sex or race. These factors have little effect on developing a healthy lifestyle. All races, all ages can have their own bangin' bodies.

4. Form and intensity are the two most important ingredients in changing your body. You must always use perfect form and work to failure on every rep, every set. If you can commit to these two things, you're on your way to changing your body.

5. Cardio is not just for women, and strength training is not just for men. Women can benefit from resistance training to build muscles. Men need cardio to burn fat. Bottom line: Both men and women must incorporate cardio and strength training.

6. Crunches do not give you a six-pack; they only make your core stronger. We all have abs, but we need to shed the fat to show them. To see your six-pack you have to shed the body fat—incorporating cardio exercises into your workout regimen and eating less are more effective ways of bringing out the six-pack.

7. What you eat is not as important as how much you eat and when you're eating it. The bottom line: You must burn off the calories to create a bangin' body.

8. You don't have to love working out. But activity is the only way to look and feel good, so you must include it in your daily lifestyle.

9. Physical education should be a requirement at all levels of school, from elementary to grad school. Being physically fit is as important as excelling academically.

10. Children will naturally crave sugar and salts because their taste buds are not as developed as adults. To try to stop them from eating sweets and salty foods is not realistic. Get them to be active and the sugar and salt won't matter.

11. Most people do not get the results they want because they do not put in enough effort. Don't stop working out when your mind tells you to stop—stop when your body tells you to stop.

12. People with a good body have trained very hard for it. Saying that race, sex or age is a factor is taking away from their hard work—and giving you an excuse.

13. It's not possible to change fat to muscle and your muscle won't turn to fat. You must build muscles and you must burn fat. Your bones do not convert to cartilage; your heart does not change into lungs.

14. Ladies, working out does not make you big. *Not* working out enough will make you big.

15. Cardio is a very effective way of burning calories, and cardio can be whatever you want it to be: basketball, swimming, dancing, skateboarding. Cardio is nothing more than simple physical activity.

16. You must work your muscles to failure on every rep of every set for every workout.

17. Protein supplements, like shakes, are not necessary as long as you're getting your protein from natural food sources.

18. You do not need steroids to look good or gain strength. Natural is safer and cheaper, and the look lasts a whole lot longer.

19. Scale weight is not important. It's your body composition, and how you look and feel, that really matters.

20. Set realistic fitness goals. Do not expect too much too soon. You didn't gain all the weight in days or weeks. Don't expect to lose it that quickly. Quick weight loss with pills or starvation diets never works in the long run—and it's dangerous.

21. You cannot change the shape of your muscles; you can change only the size. Women cannot create long, lean muscles if they don't already have them. Guys can't create a high chest if their muscles aren't shaped that way. Genetics determines the shape of your muscles, but *you* determine how to make them as defined as they can be.

22. Parents, lead by example. You cannot be inactive and expect your kids to be active and fit. They do as you do, not as you say.

23. Be honest with yourself. Police your own behavior. You know when you're making the effort and you know when you're not.

24. Stop being lazy. Take the stairs. Walk across town. Just start moving your body.

25. Video games are not a form of physical activity.

26. Stop counting calories, and just start burning them. You know when you're eating too much; adjust your workout accordingly.

27. Don't just train to look better than the average girl or guy. Always strive to be the best of the best. Just because your friend or relative is fatter than you, doesn't mean that you don't need to work out. Be the best that *you* can be. You're competing only with yourself.

28. Be patient. Do not expect to totally transform your body overnight. Like a sculptor creating a masterpiece, you can't get a bangin' body in just a few sessions. You'll get there in due time.

29. "It's not what you eat, it's what you do" is not your green light to eating more. Our motto says this: Start being more physically active, and stop focusing so much energy on food. It's your lack of physical activities that will keep you from looking and feeling your best. It's your emphasis on physical activities that will make you look *bangin'*.

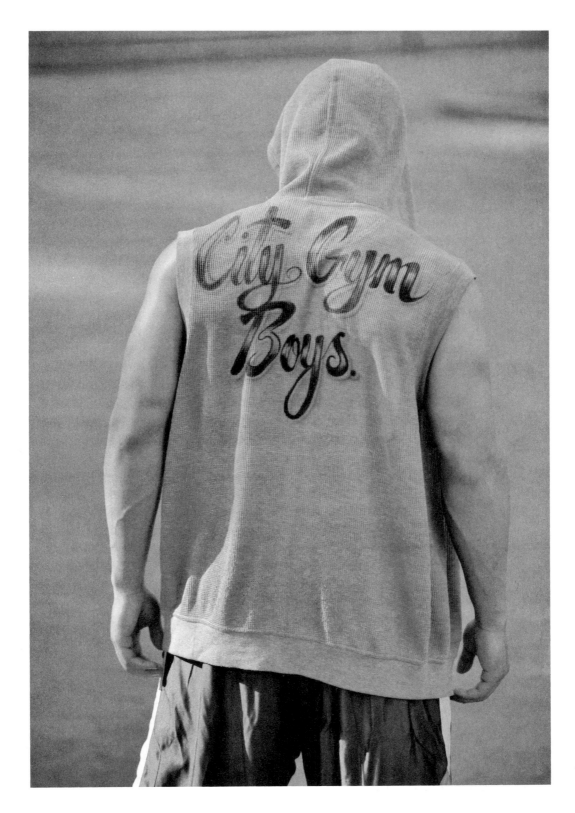

ACKNOWLEDGMENTS

First and foremost, I must thank God for giving me the vision, the strength and blessing to create City Gym Boys. My parents, for making so many sacrifices to make me the man I am today. Oprah, much thanks for inspiring me to embrace my true purpose in life and for giving me signs throughout my journey when I needed them most. My family, for always being so loving and supportive, especially my niece Michelle. CGB, past and present, for believing in the dream. I am indebted to David Barton for giving me my first personal training job and for teaching me how to be a successful trainer. Thank you to Travers Johnson, Megan Newman and everyone else at Avery for giving me this voice to speak to the world about a topic that is so passionate and real to me. I'm forever grateful, Peter Richmond, thanks for understanding and for complimenting my vision with your world-class writing skills.

We made a great team, and I look forward to many more collaborations. John Labbe, thank you for capturing the amazing images for this book. You're simply the best. Brian Mulligan, thanks for being a true visionary with this amazing book design. My legal team of Dara Onofrio and Billy Mandeville, words cannot begin to express my gratitude. Dara, much love for believing in me from the beginning of CGB and always being there for me over the years. Ann Hill and Timmy Bayly, thanks for being my true angels. Much love always. Special thanks to Jelani Medford, my friend/right-hand man, and Anthony "Top Dogg" Gittens, biomechanic specialist for assisting me on the exercise and workout chapters. You guys rock. Kian Brown, thanks for your commitment, hard work and professionalism. Francisco Perez, what can I say . . . thanks for always being a reliable friend and a dedicated team player.

Much love to my CGB supporters over the years. Your generosity is truly appreciated and will never be forgotten: Epperson, Rob Jackson, Darrin Henson, Tara Matteo, Philomena Mooney, Lynn Blank, Henry Amoroso, Rich Osler, Jason Bravo, Antoine Tempe, Pierre Cunningham, Pablo Flores, Alexis Henry, Carlton Jones, Adam Silver, Julian Watson, J's Big Gym, Deon Levingston, Fernando Natalici, Jonathan Atkin, Wayne Summerlin, Brian Amoroso, Patricia Tillery (aka Ms. T) and last but not least, our devoted and loyal CGB fans all over the world.

Always believe you can and you will. Remember failure is never an option.

RELATED READING

I hope that this book has inspired you to continue on the path to health and fitness. The below articles and websites provide information that may help you understand some of the problems you might have encountered or they may assist you in your efforts to find answers to find answers to some of your questions.

"Rising Obesity Will Coast U.S. health care $344 billion a year," *USA Today*, November 17, 2009

"Beating Obesity," *The Atlantic*, May 2010

"Record Level of Stress Found in College Freshmen," *The New York Times*, January 26, 2011

"Pressures of High School and Economy Weigh on College Freshmen," *The New York Times*, January 27, 2011

"Losing Our Way," *The New York Times*, March 25, 2011

"The Body Project: School Program Measures Obesity Right Along with Grades" *The Huffington Post*, April 4, 2011

Harper's Index, *Harper's Magazine*, September 2010

"Philadelphia School Battles Student's Bad Eating Habits, On Campus and Off," *The New York Times*, March 27, 2011

"Childhood Obesity and Self-Esteem," *The Journal of Pediatrics*, 2011

"For Obese People, Prejudice in Plain Sight," *The New York Times, March* 15, 2010

"Diabetics Confront a Tangle of Workplace Laws," *The New York Times*, December 26, 2006

"Less Active at Work, Americans Have Packed on Pounds," *The New York Times*, May 25, 2011

"The Economic Costs of Obesity," *The Brookings Institution*, September 14, 2010

"Protein-Rich Diet Helps Gorillas Keep Lean," *The New York Times*, June 3, 2011

"Quality Time, Redefined," *The New York Times*, April 29, 2011

"USU Research: Obesity Blunts Economic Prospects for Women," *The Salt Lake Tribune*, June 17, 2011

"Minority Children Face More Obesity Risks," *The Boston Globe*, March 1, 2010

"Heavy in School, Burdened for Life," *The New York Times*, June 2, 2011

"State Intervention in Life-Threatening Childhood Obesity," *The Journal of the American Medical Association*, 2011

INDEX

ABOUT THE AUTHORS

CHARLES LASALLE, founder of City Gym Boys, is an award-winning bodybuilder, certified fitness expert, motivational speaker, actor and author. Sensitive to the current obesity epidemic plaguing inner-city youth, LaSalle has directed the efforts of the City Gym Boys on spreading their fitness philosophy: "It's not what you eat, it's what you do. Start moving your bodies." The former cohost of *Fit Family* on Discovery Health and Fit TV, LaSalle believes in living his dreams. He credits his Jamaican and Cuban parents for his aggressive drive and passion to achieve. Please visit his website at www.citygymboys.com.

PETER RICHMOND has written several books, among them the *New York Times* bestseller *The Glory Game* with NFL great Frank Gifford. Richmond's work has appeared in *The New Yorker, The New York Times Magazine, Rolling Stone, GQ* and other periodicals, and in more than a dozen anthologies, including *Best American Sportswriting of the Twentieth Century*. He is currently working on a biography of basketball coach Phil Jackson.

ABOUT CITY GYM BOYS

Founded in 1997, City Gym Boys is a fitness company dedicated to mentoring inner-city youth on the lifelong benefits of fitness and exercise. Under the leadership of Charles LaSalle, it has as its urgent mission to eliminate the illnesses and conditions associated with obesity. Fifteen years after its founding, City Gym Boys has moved beyond the walls of the gym to spread its mission of shaping minds and bodies. CGB now has twenty-four members, representing more than fourteen nationalities, and it partners regularly with Dr. Mehmet Oz's HealthCorps, the American Diabetes Association and First Lady Michelle Obama's Let's Move! initiative. CGB also sponsors a long-standing weekly youth fitness program with the Boys & Girls Club of Harlem. The City Gym Boys are proof of how years of dedication, patience and physical activity can change one's body, mind and life. For more information, go to www.citygymboys.com.